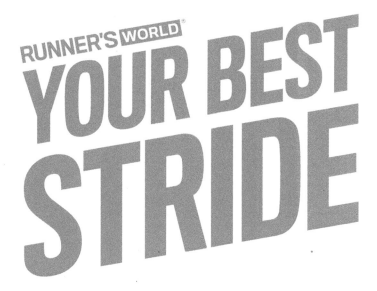

RUNNER'S WORLD®

YOUR BEST STRIDE

RUNNER'S WORLD®
YOUR BEST STRIDE

How to Optimize
Your Natural Running
Form to Run Easier,
Farther, and Faster—
With Fewer Injuries

JONATHAN BEVERLY

RODALE.

RODALE *wellness*

Live happy. Be healthy. Get inspired.

Sign up today to get exclusive access to our authors, exclusive bonuses, and the most authoritative, useful, and cutting-edge information on health, wellness, fitness, and living your life to the fullest.

Visit us online at RodaleWellness.com
Join us at RodaleWellness.com/Join

Rodale books may be purchased for business or promotional use or for special sales. For information, please write to: Trade Books/Special Markets Department, Rodale Inc., 733 Third Avenue, New York, NY 10017.

Runner's World is a registered trademark of Rodale Inc.

Printed in the United States of America

Rodale Inc. makes every effort to use acid-free ∞, recycled paper ♺.

Book design by Joanna Williams

Illustrations by Charlie Layton

Library of Congress Cataloging-in-Publication Data is on file with the publisher.

ISBN 978-1-62336-897-5 paperback

Distributed to the trade by Macmillan

4 6 8 10 9 7 5 3   paperback

RODALE.

Follow us @RodaleBooks on 🐦 📘 🅿 📷

We inspire health, healing, happiness, and love in the world. Starting with you.

To Tracy,
who continually inspires me to never settle for less than my best strides
and who has always taken the journey with me

CONTENTS

CHAPTER 1
TWO MYTHS
There is no such thing as the perfect stride that fits everyone, but you can still work to improve yours.
1

CHAPTER 2
LANDING ZONE
Foot strike, the darling of minimalism, is overrated. Why you should move your focus upward.
13

CHAPTER 3
IT'S ALL IN THE HIPS
A balanced and connected core is the key to running well.
23

CHAPTER 4
THE PERILS OF SITTING
How to reclaim your full, powerful stride
35

CHAPTER 5
REAR ENGINE
The beauty of your backside and how to build its strength
53

CHAPTER 6
HOW YOUR LAPTOP, SMARTPHONE, AND CAR ARE KILLING YOUR STRIDE
Restore your natural arm swing to improve posture and power.
73

CHAPTER 7
THE BASE
Strengthening the platform you balance on
95

CHAPTER 8
GOT RHYTHM?
The benefits—and limits—of a faster rolling stride
105

PREFACE

LIKE FLOATING ON AIR

ON A LATE-SUMMER EVENING IN 1999, I attended my first European professional track meet in Brussels, Belgium. I remember the setting sun slanting through the roof, the roar of the crowds, and the thrill of watching some of the best in the sport race. But what I remember most were the Kenyan steeplechasers.

As that event approached, several European and American runners were warming up, running along the track and taking the hurdles in typical fashion: jumping up, lightly touching the top, and pushing off. The athletes looked fit and comfortable with the challenges of the event, far more than I would be with tackling the high, sturdy hurdles of the 3,000-meter race.

Then a group of tall, thin Kenyan runners emerged. They floated along the track as if they didn't need to touch the ground, bounding over the hurdles effortlessly, like a herd of deer crossing a fence. They seemed to move in a different way than even the other world-class runners in the event. I watched in wonder at the ease with which they ran as much as at their dominance of the race.

Five years later, I was back in Brussels for the World Cross Country Championships. As competitors from around the world struggled through laps of a muddy field, one runner, Kenenisa Bekele of Ethiopia, floated in front, comfortably winning both the long (12K) and short (4K) race. More than just fitter and faster, he seemed to defy both gravity and the challenging footing of the terrain. His feet brushed the ground lightly. He accelerated smoothly and effortlessly, on demand, his legs spinning beneath a seemingly weightless body.

I've been a runner since my freshman year of high school, way back in 1977. I've had moderate success and stayed relatively injury-free. But as I watched the world's best runners, in Brussels and elsewhere, I felt like I did something entirely different than them. Instead of floating, I muscled my body along, pounding the ground and working for each forward push. Photos of me midmarathon looked like I was racewalking, particularly compared to someone like Bekele or road and cross-country champion Lornah Kiplagat, whom I watched on video and tried to emulate—with little success.

A FOOT FOCUS

Something else that caught my attention in Brussels in 2004: A blond Australian, Benita Johnson, won the women's long race over the heavily favored African runners. When I interviewed her afterward, she talked about growing up barefoot.

"I rarely wore shoes as a child," she told me the day after her surprise victory. "I grew up in the small coastal town of Mackay in Queensland, between Brisbane and Cairns. We lived outside of town, and until I went to high school in town at 13, I never even wore shoes to school. I had two brothers and one sister and we were very active; every day we were involved in sporting activities. We used to run up the sand hills on the shore—short sprints, maybe 30 seconds up the hills—then down into the ocean, then back up again."

Johnson's revelation added to my growing fascination with barefoot running. After a trip to Kenya in 2007—where I saw the fabled children running to school and at play, barefoot, free, light, and fast—I was more convinced that there was something important going on here.

I was not alone. Within the next 5 years, the entire running world became infatuated with barefoot or minimalist running. The answer, it seemed, to the question of why some runners move lightly and some plod along was to be found by paying attention to the feet.

Minimalism made sense to me. While I never became a raving barefooter, I ran barefoot strides and had the kids I coached running them. I focused on trying to land on my midfoot or forefoot and to keep my stride under my center of gravity.

Nike came out with their Free model in 2004, and they became part of my regular rotation of trainers. I tried on my first Vibram FiveFingers shoe at the 2007 Boston Marathon and started doing some training in them. I upped my use of the Vibrams after meeting Tony Post, then president and CEO of Vibram USA, at a conference in Austin, Texas, called The Running Event. One morning at the group trail run, Post, who is a solidly built, athletic man, was running comfortably in his FiveFingers. I fell in beside him, and we talked about his experience in the shoes for several miles. He was the first person I had met who treated them as running footwear, not as a training tool. Even taking into account his vested interest in broadening the shoe's appeal, Post was a true believer and a convincing advocate.

The minimalist shoes did seem to help me run quieter and lighter, although my stride and my familiar aches and pains remained largely unchanged. I particularly had troubles in my hips, hamstrings, and sacroiliac joint (tailbone).

By 2009 I ran a road 5K in a pair of Vibram FiveFingers Bikilas. Although I ran comfortably and fast in them, interestingly, a photo from the finish line of that race shows me with my forward foot toe up, about to touch down on my heel. It seemed that the shoes hadn't changed my stride much. And, while I advocated for "less shoe" among the high school runners I coached, I found that some could run well in minimal shoes but others would get hurt and instead ran better in more stable or more cushioned footwear.

Such was the experience of many, it turned out. While minimalism promised to deliver a new stride, wearing these shoes or no shoes only seemed to signal where changes were necessary. In *Running Times*, we published stories like "Are You Ready for Minimal?"—an assessment of the mobility, balance, and strengths you needed to run well in less shoe. We repeatedly reminded people of the need for time to adapt to the new mechanics.

But runners began to question the need to adapt, particularly when the new shoes didn't prevent injury but instead introduced different ones (like the metatarsal stress fracture I suffered in 2011 after doing considerable training in spikes and minimalist shoes). With the 2012 class-action lawsuit against Vibram, related to false claims in advertising that the shoes could reduce foot injuries and strengthen foot muscles, the tide had completely turned. After lifting the hero of minimalism (Vibram) onto a godlike pedestal, the running world dragged it to the edge of town and stoned it to death. More than 150,000—claimants for a piece of the Vibram settlement—threw stones. The minimalist movement was dead.

As shoe companies began to go back to more cushioned and more controlling shoes, and minimalism became a dirty word, one question hung out there unanswered, "How should we then run?" Throwing out our shoes (or at least our heel lifts and medial posts) may not be the answer, but we seemed to have thrown out the baby with the bathwater. Minimalism had gone too far—becoming a religion with rules and levels of commitment—and it had offered the wrong solution: different shoes. But at its core was the idea that we could run better.

HOW SHOULD WE THEN RUN?

It was in this context, in the fall of 2013, that I set out to discover if, in a postminimalist world, I could find any consensus among athletes, coaches, physical therapists, podiatrists, biomechanists, and form gurus about what is good form and how to improve it.

For 3 months, I immersed myself in research about running form. Every other day I spoke with another expert. I read research reports, articles, and books. And I tried out everything I heard and read. The result in the magazine was a feature story called, "It's All in the Hips."

The result for me was learning more about how I move than I had in my previous 50 years. I learned how far off balance my default posture was and marveled at how tall and comfortable I felt in "neutral." I found myself correcting my balance any time I was standing and began playing with what coach Bobby McGee calls "dynamic balance," leaning out from neutral so that I needed force under my toes to stay upright. From there I learned to fall into motion effortlessly, rather than reaching a leg out and pulling myself forward.

I felt the rotation necessary to get my hips in neutral after doing one of the tests recommended by Jay Dicharry, biomechanics researcher, physical therapist, and director of the REP Biomechanics Lab in Bend, Oregon—a test, incidentally, that had appeared in the magazine before, but I confess I had never tried, not thinking I had to work on posture. I learned how to do a squat properly for the first time, feeling it all in my butt, not in my quads and knees.

At The Running Event conference in Austin that December, I was kicked in the butt—repeatedly—by exercise therapist/rehab specialist Laura Bergmann as she tried to get me in the proper position to do a side-leg lift. When she did, I felt the correct muscles working for the first time and realized I had never worked them properly.

I watched the video of Robby Andrews winning the 2011 NCAA 800-meter race and noted, as Dicharry pointed out, how most of the field rotated their pelvis and arched their back as they fatigued, and how the three who didn't medaled. I started noting hip position changing with fatigue in other runners—and in me.

Using coach Tom Miller's posture bar, a PVC pipe, I felt how far back my arms should be driving behind my torso. Then I needed Bergmann's help to open up my shoulders in order to swing freely in that posture and to keep my arms driving back that far during my runs.

One day, during a 400-meter repeat, things came together.

As I crested the slight grade on the dirt road and pushed toward the clump of bushes that marked the finish of that segment, I noticed something different. Usually I'd start to wallow in the effort at this point, my legs feeling like Silly Putty as they dragged the dead weight of my torso through the final meters.

This day, however, my legs were spinning in a perfect, powerful gear. My hips felt locked in, stable, and connected, transferring energy seamlessly to my spine like a well-tuned carbon-fiber bike frame. My body felt compact, balanced, and flying. I didn't have to flail and strive to finish the repeat—all I had to do was maintain my turnover.

It was what Rob Conenello, DPM, sports podiatrist, runner, and form expert, calls the "aha moment"—the instant it clicks and you feel for yourself what people like Conenello are talking about in terms of posture, hip rotation, hip extension, glute activation, and other elements of an effective stride.

What surprised me, given my years of running, was how much I didn't know and how much I could still improve. True, I've known that I wasn't like Kenenisa, but I've had a form that works well enough to have run, quite successfully, for a lifetime.

I've always seen myself as a smooth, efficient runner. How did I get to this point without knowing how to really use my glutes? One consolation came from seeing that even runners in top groups, runners of the caliber of Deena Kastor, Meb Keflezighi, and Mo Farah have to continually work on improving how they move.

A PROCESS, NOT A PROBLEM

More than that, however, I began to see that the process of having good form, or more accurately, of moving more effectively, is not something you are born being able to do or not do, nor is it simply a matter of good or bad movement habits like how your foot lands. Running well requires an effective range of motion in your limbs and specific strengths. Most of the habits of our day-to-day lives work against us in these areas, limiting our mobility, balance, and appropriate strength, to the extent that whole muscle groups get shut off and we lose the ability to move the way we did when we were 3 or 4 years old.

There are many reasons African runners move so beautifully and powerfully. One big one stems from their upbringing and lifestyle. In a country without the "conveniences" we take for granted, they walk and run for transportation, stand more than they sit, and work and play in highly physical ways as a daily part of life: carrying tools, groceries, or whatever they need to transport; hoeing gardens; building by hand; squatting; playing soccer; and not sitting in a chair hunched over a computer when not wrapped around a smartphone.

My experience is, of course, only the experiment of one, but I can report that learning to feel the position of my hips, activate my glutes, and play with my balance has transformed how I move. I feel better while running and all day long. My running has been smoother, easier, and injury-free, even with increased miles and as a master. After last year's Fourth of July race I wrote down, "One of the easiest 5Ks muscularly I can remember." A year later, I ran an age-graded PR, feeling smoother than ever. At an international group trail run, where I was one of the oldest participants, I was pleased to be told I had a light, bouncy stride.

I keep learning not only how much I need to continue working at the elements I focused on in 2013, but also how other parts of my body are affected by 21st century lifestyles and conveniences—shoulders, neck, feet. I jumped into a treadmill video analysis at a conference in December 2015 and discovered that I still needed work in all the same areas of posture, hips, shoulders, and overstriding. I'm coming to peace with the fact that this isn't something I can focus on once and have solved. I need to incorporate habitual corrective exercises into my daily routines or else lose—all too quickly—the gains I've made.

I know improving my form hasn't worked and won't work magic: I still have to do the miles, the hills, and the speed work to get fit enough to race well. And it requires fairly constant mindfulness, which can mess with the relaxing, therapeutic side of running. But it has been worth it to feel lighter, smoother, and younger—not to mention pain-free—on the run.

This book is a compilation of what I've learned. Little to none of it is original—it draws from the expertise of many scientists, physicians, and coaches—but I hope the presentation and organization in this format will help you to pay attention, understand better how and why you move the way you do, incorporate new habits into your routine, and, in the end, run easier and better.

INTRODUCTION

WHO NEEDS THIS BOOK?

YOUR RUNNING STYLE IS MUCH like your voice. Every person has a distinct sound based on his or her physical characteristics, habits, and upbringing. Most people don't think much about how their voice sounds, know what makes it sound that way, or have any clue how to change it if they wanted to.

Some voices are high-pitched, while others are deep. Some voices have a nasal overtone, maybe only temporarily because of a cold, or maybe more permanently out of habit or the shape of throat and nasal passages. Some have accents, based on early influences; one might linger on long vowels, while another might clip or roll his or her *r*'s. As long as we can communicate, each voice works.

There are times, however, when you need to pay attention to your voice. If your speech pattern varies so far from the norm that it can't be understood, you need to change it. You need speech therapy or an accent-reduction class, where you'll learn more about how the throat, tongue, and lips form sounds and how you can alter them. And you'll practice new patterns until they become reproducible and, eventually, your new habit.

Alternatively, if you want to excel with your voice, such as using it to be a singer, public speaker, actor, or broadcaster, you will likely need to work to make it more effective. Some just want to get a bit better, like learning to project to perform in the school play. Some make it their profession: Entire university degrees are based upon improving the quality and effectiveness of your voice. You can buy books, get instructional DVDs, and hire coaches to help you sound better for your chosen field.

Similarly, every runner has a stride signature based around his or her unique characteristics. It usually develops without thought or training, and most people don't think about how it looks, why it works the way it does, or how to change it. When they are ready to run, they are able to run.

ARE YOUR WHEELS FALLING OFF?

As with a voice that doesn't communicate, however, runners need to change their stride if it doesn't function properly. Runners who are chronically injured need to figure out why. Athlete, coach, and assistant professor of kinesiology at Southeastern Louisiana University Ryan Green, PhD, says, "Bad running injures people. Our bodies have the capacity to run healthy."

"If you are running well without injury or problem, then why fix something that isn't broken?" says Harvard professor and running movement researcher Daniel Lieberman, PhD. "But if you are getting injured on a regular basis, why wouldn't you look at your form? Sometimes injuries are the result of simply too much too fast, and thus not allowing the body to adapt. Sometimes they are caused by weaknesses (e.g., weak abductors), but sometimes they are caused by poor running form."

Lieberman points out that tibial stress syndrome, which starts as shin splints, is caused by the impact stresses of overstriding. The pain of shin splints is a signal that you are doing something wrong. "Rather than treat the symptom, why not fix the problem? That involves changing one's form."

Sometimes you may want to fix something before it breaks. "You can run with crappy form for a very long time," says mobility expert Brad Cox. But if you start to increase your miles, want to get faster, or simply are getting older, ineffective mechanics can start to haunt you. "Most people only use pain as a reason that they start looking for anything else," Cox says. Before the pain, he recommends that you need to check on your mechanics and mobility regularly.

BE YOUR BEST YOU

Thinking this way leads to a second reason to consider form. Like the opera singer or network anchor who spends years tuning her voice, runners who want to be their best leave no stone unturned, including their form, even if they function fairly well now. "Running is a skill," says Lieberman. "Learning a skill means training one's motor patterns." Elite runners work on every element of this skill every day.

"I think every runner should be concerned with form," says Scott Simmons, coach of the American Distance Project. He clarifies, though, that it is not about changing to match a certain ideal, but about paying attention to biomechanics, "trying to identify an individual's inefficiencies with mobility, range of motion, specific strength, and symmetry."

Over the years of covering top athletes as editor in chief of

Running Times, I increasingly learned that all of them—from high school champions to world record holders—don't rely simply on running to build their dominance. While you'll rarely find a Kenyan or Ethiopian runner inside a weight room, you will see them doing extensive drills and ancillary exercises to improve their strength, agility, explosive power, and speed. The same is true if you visit a collegiate practice or drop in on an elite marathoner like Shalane Flanagan or Meb Keflezighi.

You may wonder why I'm talking about weights and drills; isn't this a book on form? I'm sorry to tell you that most of what is recommended in the pages to come involves work—stretches, exercises, foam rolling, and more—not simply cuing new patterns or changing your shoes.

I won't overpromise anything. Focusing on form takes effort and time—there are no simple, quick fixes that will magically make you better. And progress may not be very visible. But the outcome, says Irish performance scientist John Kiely, is that "you will be a more robust athlete. More resilient." Being a more resilient runner will allow you to run longer and train harder, with less risk of injury.

You may find this book useful if:

❯ You want to run more smoothly and effectively.

❯ You have tried and failed to change your stride or are not interested in adopting a new stride pattern based on some sort of "ideal" form.

❯ You have reached a performance plateau and would like to find ways to become faster and more efficient.

❯ You have small but persistent injuries or pains associated with running that have not been cured by traditional medicine or changes in shoes.

> You have pains that appear when you reach a certain volume of training, no matter how gradually you ramp up to it.

> You are getting older—either old enough to start feeling the effects of imbalances and lack of mobility, or old enough to know that you will run into problems someday soon and you want to extend your running life.

> You are confused by all the talk about form retraining—particularly now that minimalism has been largely abandoned and research gives us seemingly contradictory information about shoes, stride, injuries, and performance.

> You want to learn more about how your body works so you can better assess and optimize your form during running.

Plus:

> Like most of us in the modern world, you live in a society where walking or running is not the primary form of transportation.

> You spend the majority of your daily hours sitting: at a desk, driving, in a living room watching TV, or reading. You rarely perform physical labor that involves your whole body: lifting, pushing, bending, or reaching.

You probably don't need the book if:

> You live in a rural setting in a developing country like Kenya and have maintained a traditional, preindustrial lifestyle since youth.

> You run pain-free, at the pace you want to, and are not getting older.

1
TWO MYTHS

THERE IS NO SUCH THING AS THE PERFECT
STRIDE THAT FITS EVERYONE, BUT YOU CAN
STILL WORK TO IMPROVE YOURS.

ANY RUNNER WHO DIVES INTO the subject of running form quickly
finds it is a thorny topic. Looking for simple advice, you discover
opposing camps, separated not just by nuances like scheduling
or selection of workouts, but in their beliefs regarding what is
true and how we should then live. That sounds almost religious,
and it can often feel that way, with different groups taking on
the fervor of cults, complete with gurus, tenets of belief, and
unique rituals.

Different camps exist, and thrive, because we don't know
enough to prove one is true. Research is often limited and contradictory. Every camp can produce testimonials of how its program saved this or that individual's running life. And each also
has detractors who failed to reach the promised land. It is therefore left to each runner to find what works for her or him—and
different runners find success with different approaches.

We do know enough, however, to dispel two persistent myths.
One is that there exists a perfect running form that we all should

emulate. The other, opposite, myth is that however we move is just the way we are—by birth, upbringing, or both—and nothing we do can change that. These two myths are not exclusive. Many believe both: that there is a perfect form but they weren't gifted with it and can't do anything about it.

These myths tend to demoralize and paralyze runners. Trying to emulate Kenenisa Bekele's form, or whatever is perceived as "perfection," more often than not fails. Even if you are successful at changing your habits, it often doesn't make you faster, smoother, or injury-free.

Believing that you were born a certain way robs you of any incentive to improve. "That's just the way I am," is the only possible response, for better or worse. With that outlook, all you can do is accept your limitations, train to become fitter, and try to find shoes that fit your stride type and support your weaknesses. The idea that shoes can solve all ills is a third, perhaps even more pervasive, myth that I'll take up later in the book.

These myths are persistent because they all hold a bit of truth.

THE PERFECT RUNNING MACHINE

It's easy to see the logic of those who argue for a perfect form: If humans are meant to run, there must be a natural, optimal way to do it. We all have the same parts. We're all fighting the same forces of gravity, friction, and wind resistance.

Where should we look to find what that form looks like? An obvious place would seem to be those who run faster over distance than anyone else in the world today: the East Africans.

If you stand on the side of Commonwealth Avenue in Boston, Massachusetts, on the third Monday in April you can watch the world's best runners go by. After 22 miles they are still flowing quickly down the road, moving lightly and smoothly, with a spring in their step.

Compare these runners to the rest of the pack, and you'll see that those up front share several elements of form, whereas the form of those behind falls apart in various ways. To paraphrase Leo Tolstoy's quote about families: All good runners resemble one another; each inefficient runner is inefficient in his or her own way. If we could run exactly like those frontrunners, it seems obvious that we would move faster, smoother, and more efficiently. That is a big if, for many reasons.

STRIDE SIGNATURE

Look more closely at that lead pack and you'll note that, despite the shared effortlessness, each of these very efficient runners has his or her own unique style. Each has individual movement patterns that create a running signature. It may be a head bob, one arm that swings wide, or feet that pinwheel at the back of the stride.

We've all seen these signatures before. If I am meeting a running friend in a busy venue like New York's Central Park or Boston's Charles River, or if I'm watching for someone in the throng of a marathon field, I don't need to wait to see facial features to recognize him or her. A runner's stride identifies him from a mile away, even amid a sea of other runners.

In 2012, Brigham Young University biomechanist Iain Hunter, PhD, closely examined the foot strike of runners in the Olympic Trials and found a wide variety in their landing location and angles. Even these, the best runners in the country, running on a track—a perfectly groomed surface conducive to a machine-like consistency—differed significantly from one another.

Former Olympian and coach Lee Troop isn't at all surprised. "No one is born with a 100 percent perfect body," Troop says. "Everyone of us has some deficiency somewhere. As we grow and morph, our bodies become accustomed to it. If you look at the Olympic [Marathon] start, you see 100 different runners that all have different form, different styles."

John Kiely, senior lecturer in Elite Performance at the Institute of Coaching and Performance, University of Central Lancashire, United Kingdom, explains that this variability is part of the genius of the human body. Unlike a machine, made of identical parts moving in identical pathways, our bodies are each different from one another and even variable individually: No one is perfectly symmetrical.

"Multiple dimensions of running architecture—snugness of bones within sockets, springiness of tendons, rigidity of feet, geometry of muscles—differ between individuals, sometimes subtly, sometimes dramatically," Kiely explains. "There is a right template for you. There isn't a right template for all of us."

Rather than trying to follow one path, like a machine would, and failing to perform because of these anomalies, the body instead adapts its movement patterns to optimize the pathways its own architecture allows. Kiely says, "We learn to run in ways that accommodate these mismatched parts, thanks to a pervasive aspect of human biology: plasticity, our capacity to reshape neural and biological structures in response to repeated practice."

In other words, the way we each learn to run is unique to our specific bodies. Sports podiatrist and runner Paul Langer, DPM, says, "Every person has a unique movement pattern, so you can't really make blanket statements about what is bad running form or good running form for any given person. You really can't try to get everybody to run the same."

PREFERRED MOVEMENT PATH

Your body not only creates your own style, but it also optimizes that style to use the least amount of energy. University of Calgary biomechanist Benno Nigg, PhD, calls the resulting pattern your "preferred movement path." In studies, Nigg and colleagues found that most runners will maintain this preferred path even when wearing shoes or inserts designed to alter or control the motion of their stride. Other studies, ranging from the 1982 work of early running researcher Peter Cavanagh, PhD, on self-chosen stride lengths published in *Medicine and Science in Sports and Exercise,* to a 2005 study at Colorado State University on an attempt to retrain runners' gait, show that runners tend to be most efficient using this "preferred pattern."

"Mammals move in a way that is both metabolically efficient and least painful," says Langer. "Anything that deviates from that preferred movement pattern increases metabolic costs." Langer and fellow podiatrist Rob Conenello, DPM, say that unless a runner is having difficulties, they don't advise trying to change his or her form to match a preconceived ideal.

"I think it's important to recognize that everyone has a fairly unique 'movement signature,'" says David McHenry, DPT, a physical therapist and strength coach for elite runners including athletes at Nike's Oregon Project. "I think a goal of changing form is first starting with the realization that the further away from their natural movement signature you are trying to take someone, the more unlikely you will make the sustainable change that you are going for."

McHenry cites Mo Farah and Galen Rupp, two runners he has worked with, as examples. "Both are clearly two of the best and most consistent distance runners in the world over the past

4 years," McHenry says. "And both have very different running styles. We don't try to make Mo run like Galen and [we] don't try to make Galen run like Mo."

The way we run is unique to our bodies and our experience. I can no more run like Kenenisa Bekele than he could run like me (not that he would want to). Bottom line: There is no "perfect" form, no "one-size-fits-all" recommendation.

But if stride is ingrained and personal—if it not only can't be changed but also shouldn't be messed with—what is the purpose of this book?

Limits to the Preferred Movement Path

The problem with "I'm just the way I am" is that we aren't. We aren't who we are meant to be, or who we once were. At one point in our lives, yes, most of us moved without restriction—when we were very young.

Watch a 4-year-old girl run barefoot across a lawn and marvel at the smooth effortlessness. When she wants to get from one side of the playground to the other quickly, she doesn't strain or lumber into a run, she simply levitates and lightly dances there. Note, as well, that she runs much like the others of her age cavorting around her. Like the world-class elites at the front of the marathon, their large movement patterns are all similar, with small, individual variations.

The similarities among those who run well reflects that while each individual runs best in the way his or her body wants to move, some elements of style are universal to the human form and its anatomy. If we start to deviate from these key movement patterns, our bodies will still find a way to run, but the motion paths and muscles recruited will be less efficient, and we'll become more prone to injury.

Yes, we have a preferred path, but that path is based not only on the geometries and motion preferences of our bodies at birth, but also on the parameters of our lifestyles and training. And our lives are not generally conducive to maintaining the flexibility, posture, balance, and strengths that allow for the best movement patterns for our bodies.

This is the theme of Harvard professor Daniel Lieberman's book, *The Story of the Human Body*, namely, that cultural and environmental changes in our lifestyles have created mismatches between what our bodies do well and what we ask them to do day by day. "We enjoy rest and relaxation, but our bodies are still those of endurance athletes evolved to walk many miles a day and often run, as well as dig, climb, and carry," Lieberman writes. "We love many comforts, but we are not well adapted to spend our days indoors in chairs, wearing supportive shoes, staring at books or screens for hours on end."

The resulting "mismatch diseases"—unintended consequences of too much comfort—include many of the injuries we ascribe to shoes or poor form. Lieberman details, for example, how the comfort of sitting in a chair can lead to muscle atrophy and shortened muscles, creating postural weakness and imbalances.

"We are not living the lives our bodies were designed for—in terms of the air we breathe, the food we eat, and our activity levels," says Irene Davis, PhD, a professor at Harvard Medical School and the director of the Spaulding National Running Center. "I believe this extends to the way we are running today. There is a very high incidence of injuries doing something that we evolved to do. That would be like a fish getting fin injuries from swimming."

Those who see contextual compromises in form don't throw out the individuality of each runner's stride. "I have a high level of respect for preferred movement patterns," says Langer, "but sometimes a movement pattern may be faulty because [a runner has] a core muscle imbalance or maybe poor range of motion in their hip flexors."

Nigg maintains that the self-chosen, preferred movement path is always close to optimal in terms of energy use. Yet he makes clear that our paths are not static or always ideal. "There's a difference in the preferred movement path that you could have ever and the preferred movement path that you can have now," Nigg says. "Now you have muscles that are not strong enough and muscles that are too strong. In that situation your preferred movement path is different than the situation where you are completely trained and all your muscles are trained."

Nigg gives the example of a study he conducted that compared individuals with weak and strong ankle muscles. Those with weak small muscles around the ankle had to recruit big muscles up the calf through the Achilles tendon to create stability. Those large muscles are wired for power, not stability—so they used much more energy to accomplish the task, even while doing it poorly. "So this preferred pattern is not ideal. If you want to win a championship, that is a stupid thing to have," Nigg says. "But at the moment, that is what you have."

It makes no sense for a runner in this situation to claim that this is just the way he or she is. The current preferred path isn't based around a genetic difference but a trainable, changeable characteristic. So, "you work on small muscles, make them stronger," says Nigg. "Then you have a preferred movement path that is much better."

RELEASING THE NATURAL FLOW

We can think of the preferred movement path like water flowing down a mountainside. Each mountain is unique, so the specific route will vary as the water takes the path of least resistance down the mountainside's contours. It would take considerable wasteful effort to redirect water that is flowing down one mountainside so that its path matches the path on another mountain. To match it exactly, you would have to restructure the entire mountain so that every ridge and valley resembled the other—an idea that gets even more absurd when applying this analogy to the human body.

But if one stream encountered a dam that backed it up and made it swirl in an eddy before proceeding down, it would be clear that the dam was altering the preferred path of water down that mountainside. Clearing the dam so that the stream flowed unhindered down the entire route would make it more efficient, without trying to change the mountain to something it isn't.

When it comes to running, we all have dams that can keep us from moving in our natural paths. Each individual has his or her own physical limitations. Some of them are unique and/or significant enough to need professional medical assistance. Some problems, however, are systemic to the 21st-century lifestyle. Within a few short years, that 4-year-old we saw running smoothly across the lawn will be sitting at a desk for far more of the day than she will be running around, jumping, climbing, digging, or carrying. Soon she will be hunched over a laptop or a cell phone. At age 16, she'll likely start driving, adding to her sitting and forward-reaching time.

All of these habits restrict our mobility, create imbalances, and weaken key muscle groups. And those restrictions and weaknesses make us run less than optimally.

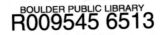

Running better, however, requires more than some cues to focus on during the run. We don't stride imperfectly because we learned poor habits. "A poor movement pattern is usually a symptom of something else," podiatrist Langer says.

Kiely, arguing from the perspective of both researcher and coach, agrees. "Technical change is very hard," Kiely says. "If you want to implement technical change, telling someone to do something different is practically useless, if not detrimental."

If there are obstructions that are causing damage or inefficiencies, we need to change more than the instructions coming from the brain. "Let's change elements of the system," Kiely says. "Give something more strength, improve balance, coordination, or proprioception. Let's in some way change the system we are controlling, then let's recalibrate the controller with the controlling system."

That controlling system will still be you, the highly skilled organism that adapts to the parameters your body gives it. The goal is to give it a better set of parameters.

"I do not think there is one way to run," says Brad Cox, coach, mobility specialist, and cofounder of the educational company Acumobility. "But, if you can identify some of the things life has thrown at you that are affecting you—and can clean them up— you can dramatically improve and enjoy running far more."

"The goal is to run like *you*, but a better you," says McHenry.

This is what you'll find in the pages to come: how to identify and clear the dams to let the water flow as it once did—or as close as we can, with aging bodies affected by years of sitting, hunching, and getting stiff and lazy. It isn't about adopting a set of beliefs, joining a particular camp, or even matching a type of running form. It isn't about buying the right shoes. It is about rediscovering the best you: your best stride.

This book doesn't try to be exhaustive regarding possible stride problems or ways of working on them. Instead, I've tried to identify the essential, most universal elements and present a few ways you can begin working to improve. And I'll try to provide some help in finding the motivation, feedback, and patterns that will allow you to perform the work necessary to transform into the best possible runner you can be.

2
LANDING ZONE

FOOT STRIKE, THE DARLING OF MINIMALISM, IS OVERRATED. WHY YOU SHOULD MOVE YOUR FOCUS UPWARD.

WATCH A VIDEO OF KENENISA Bekele winning a 5,000-meter or 10,000-meter race, or, just last year, the Berlin Marathon, and it quickly becomes apparent that he is doing something different than what most of us do every day. Bekele and the majority of the world-class pack running with him float around the track, hardly seeming to touch it. They move smoothly, softly, with great balance.

We want to run like them, rather than pounding the ground, pulling through each step to power ourselves forward. What element of their stride creates the difference, we wonder? Where should we look?

For many years we were told to focus on their feet. Elite runners are different, form experts said, because they land on their midfoot or forefoot, and we should do the same to run smoother, faster, and with fewer injuries. A few years ago, during the height of the minimalism craze, where your foot makes contact with the ground became a litmus test of one's running prowess. Among some runners, the label "heel-striker" attained the stigma of "learning impaired."

When the masses tried to change, however, the results were mixed. Many of those who adopted a forefoot strike and the minimalist shoes that accompanied the movement didn't see an improvement in times and continued to get injured. So much so that the movement—and the shoes—have all but passed. But the question of proper or better form remains. Is there any reason to try to change your landing?

MISPLACED FOCUS

A wide range of experts—from kinesiologists to physical therapists, orthopedists to coaches—agree that the extreme emphasis the running world has put on foot strike was misplaced. Daniel Lieberman, PhD, the Harvard scientist who, with Utah biologist Dennis Bramble, PhD, gave scientific credence to minimalism with his seminal 2010 "Born to Run" article in *Nature*, says, "Frankly, when we published that paper, I never expected everyone to obsess about it as much as they did. Had I realized that, I would have added a sentence to the effect that while foot strike is important, there are many other important aspects of form as well."

"Is it bad to land on the heel?" asks biomechanics researcher Benno Nigg, who has been studying shoes and stride for 50 years. "There is no evidence whatsoever that that is a fact."

Grant Robison, retired elite runner and coach whose Good Form Running program was adopted by shoe giant New Balance to educate runners on how to move into the company's Minimus line, says that while teaching runners to land on the midfoot was an emphasis a few years ago, he now considers it the least important of the four points he teaches: posture, midfoot, cadence, and lean. "I draw people's attention to it, showing that if you can use more of your foot, things don't get stressed as much, but then I kind of let that be," Robison says.

"Foot strike is overemphasized," says Jeff Gaudette, former elite athlete and owner/head coach of RunnersConnect, an online platform through which he's coached thousands of runners, including a special course on form featuring many of the sport's leading experts. "It is not critically important. If everything else is solid, foot strike is going to take care of itself."

Jay Dicharry, biomechanics researcher, physical therapist, and director of the REP Biomechanics Lab in Bend, Oregon, agrees that foot strike is an effect, not a cause. "Certainly foot strike is getting way too much attention," he says.

He's measured heel-strikers who touch down with zero force and forefoot strikers who pound the ground. "I'm not a fan of telling someone to land on a certain spot on their foot," Dicharry says. "Landing on the forefoot doesn't fix everything."

CONFUSING CONCLUSIONS

What caused this change in focus away from the forefoot? At least two factors can be credited for the shift. First, when science caught up with the trends, conducting controlled studies on stresses and tracking injury rates, the results were far from unanimous. On the contrary, the results were often contradictory and confusing.

Several studies have shown that those who run faster do tend to land on their midfoot or forefoot more often than those farther back in the pack. These include a 1987 study by Nigg's group, one conducted in 1996 out of the University of Vermont, and a 2013 George Washington University study of Kenyan barefoot runners. But not all fast runners do. A 2007 study by the Laboratory of Exercise Science at Ryukoku University in Japan revealed that more than half of those at the very front of a half marathon (running as fast as 5 minutes/mile) touched down with their heel. Even the 2012 NCAA cross-country champion, Kenyan Kennedy Kithuka, running for Texas Tech, was a noticeable heel-striker.

More significantly, studies failed to prove the claims that forefoot striking was more economical or reduced injury. A 2012 study conducted by the running biomechanics lab at the University of Massachusetts, for example, found no difference in economy between heel- and forefoot strikers. The study suggested that heel striking might actually be more economical because, when the runners were asked to switch styles, only a few of those who switched to forefoot were more economical, but more than half of those who usually touched down on their forefoot ran more efficiently on their heels. Head researcher Allison Gruber, PhD, concluded, "These results suggest that running with a [rearfoot] pattern might confer benefits in endurance events in both habitual [rearfoot] and [forefoot] runners. Moreover, our findings do not support previous recommendations that habitual [rearfoot] runners should switch to a [forefoot] pattern to gain a performance advantage."

A 2016 overview of studies, published in *Physical Therapy Reviews*, cited one study that showed that midfoot and forefoot strikers were more economical than heel-strikers, one showing the reverse, and three revealing no difference in economy. The authors concluded, "The reviewed studies collectively suggest that foot strike pattern alone is not a determinant of running economy."

Echoing what we discussed in the previous chapter, foot strike appears to be one of those factors that is determined and shaped by the body selecting the most economical path given each runner's individual physiology. Australian podiatry professor and clinician Craig Payne writes in his *Running Research Junkie* blog, "As all our faces and other anatomical features vary, so do the joints' surface orientation and joint axis orientation vary which will affect the lever arms that tendons have. . . . That variation in lever arms will affect how hard a muscle needs to work . . . and the energy return from stored energy (i.e., economy). For some that will be heel striking, for others that will be midfoot striking, and for others that will be forefoot striking."

Simon Bartold, podiatrist, biomechanics researcher, and consultant for Salomon, says this more succinctly: "There is no best way to run. You are going to be who you are going to be."

But what about injury? Here again, studies are frustratingly contradictory. A 2012 retrospective study on collegiate distance runners showed that heel-strikers had roughly double the number of injuries than forefoot strikers did. Several other studies of large groups of recreational runners, however, revealed no correlation between foot-strike patterns and injury. One of the largest studies, presented at the 2014 American College of Sports Medicine annual meeting, looked at 1,027 soldiers and found that heel-strikers and forefoot strikers reported the same amount of injuries.

What forefoot striking does do is change the location where running stresses are applied. In 2015, Nigg wrote in *Footwear Science*, "It is known that certain structures are more loaded in forefoot landing and others more in heel landing. To use external ground reaction forces and lower leg kinematics [motions and forces] to support the claim that forefoot landing will possibly produce fewer injuries is, in our view, inappropriate."

Talking with Nigg, he echoes this, pointing out that much higher forces—4 or 5 times as much—are applied to the ankle when you land on your forefoot. He also dispels the myth that a heel strike is inherently worse for your knees and hips.

"All these things float around in the running population," Nigg says. "If you run landing on the heel, you have a shock in the knee and shock in [the] hip joint that much bigger—not true." His research shows that our system of muscles, interacting with vibrations, attenuates the shocks and adapts to whatever touchdown or cushioning it is given.

Whatever the mechanism, all of the researchers and physicians I interviewed agree that a change won't eliminate stresses that cause injury. "Run barefoot or minimalist, you're going to reduce load at the knee, and [you're] going to increase load at the Achilles tendon," says Bartold. "You cannot create or destroy load, you can only shift it, can only move it—it has to go somewhere."

This doesn't mean that changing how you land might not help you avoid injury if you need to shift forces away from a weak area. It does mean, however, that forefoot striking isn't the answer for everyone.

"Each running technique will have different biomechanical effects and different injury risk profiles," Payne writes.

UNINTENDED RESULTS

In addition to the inconclusive scientific evidence, the call for people to change their foot strike just by thinking about it has had unintended and often negative results. Runners tend to force a contrived, prancing gait that is as ineffective in producing speed as it is at reducing injury.

"I have learned over the years that the worst thing to tell anyone is to forefoot strike," Lieberman says. "If you tell people to forefoot strike, they often overdo it and land on their toes like a ballerina. Landing like that is probably a fast track to getting calf muscle damage and Achilles [injuries]."

Other experts agree that you can't get to where you're going that way. From coaches to medical professionals, they say some variation of the same line.

Robison says he no longer points out foot strike to someone on the run. "I feel that would be more confusing than help[ful]," he says. "I worked with one high school girl whom somebody sometime had obviously told to run on her forefoot. She was way up on her toes and had suffered three broken metatarsals [as a result]."

"I will never, ever, ever tell somebody to think about where their foot is hitting the ground," says physical therapist and form researcher Abby Douek of Run Raleigh Physical Therapy. "It doesn't end well. It ends up looking like a train wreck."

While some ended up messing up their stride, for most, it seems that trying to change their foot strike didn't really have any effect at all. Recent research by Martyn Shorten, PhD, head of the Portland, Oregon–based research lab BioMechanica, and others, such as reported in a 2012 study out of the Medical College of Wisconsin, show that the vast majority of runners, even those who think of and identify themselves as midfoot or forefoot strikers, actually land on their heels.

A VARIABLE AND SMOOTH LANDING

Part of the problem is that we've set up foot strike as a defining, unchangeable characteristic of the stride, when in fact it is variable and changes in different situations. In a surprising passage from biology professor and blogger Peter Larson's 2012 book, *Tread Lightly*, Lieberman says, "I think everybody does everything. This idea that you're just a forefoot striker, or just a midfoot striker, or just a heel-striker, is bizarre. Variation is what biology is all about." Lieberman points out that foot strike is dependent on many variables: speed, terrain, how much you've warmed up, footwear, and fatigue. "Why do people have to do just one thing?" he says. In this perspective, foot strike may be more like whether a tennis player chooses to use a backhand or forehand, rather than whether she is right- or left-handed.

The term *strike* is another part of the problem when we talk about landing. It implies a hard impact and carries with it connotations of thumping and injury. "It is questionable whether foot contact events even qualify as 'impacts,'" says Shorten. In the context of other forces involved in running, Shorten says, "The loads are very low magnitude, low frequency, and necessary for bone health—so what's the problem?"

You can also make contact with the ground very differently no matter which part of the foot is leading. "There is a forefoot impact that can be as big as or bigger than that in the heel," Shorten says. Landing on the heel doesn't necessarily mean pounding. Many who touch down with the heel kiss the ground lightly. "The rolling transition from heel to flat forefoot is a very gentle way of contacting the ground—a soft landing," Shorten says.

Rather than the place on the foot where you land, it seems what is happening with your leg motion and body mass at the moment you touch down is more important. What the scientists are observing and coaches are trying to create by encouraging a forefoot strike is a stride that touches lightly without braking and flows smoothly.

Given the ambivalent effects of different landing styles, coach and exercise scientist Steve Magness writes in his *Science of Run-*

ning blog, "Perhaps we should consider looking at foot strike in terms of where it occurs in relation to your center of mass, instead of where it occurs on the foot."

"It's *not* rearfoot or midfoot or forefoot that matters," Dicharry says. "It's where the foot contacts in relation to the body's center of mass."

Bobby McGee, the Boulder-based running coach, talks about the landing angle of the shin, which reflects the direction in which forces are being applied. Canadian physiotherapist Blaise Dubois also talks about shin angles and distinguishes a hard, negative heel strike from an effective "proprioceptive heel strike" in which "the foot flattens smoothly as soon as it hits the ground" and where it "doesn't involve a strong braking phase or brutal impact force."

But creating such a landing just by thinking about it is as futile as trying to change your foot strike. Even if you could sense it accurately, it is close to impossible to modify it by focusing on it. The focus is still in the wrong place.

3
IT'S ALL IN THE HIPS

A BALANCED AND CONNECTED CORE IS THE KEY TO RUNNING WELL.

THE MINIMALIST MOVEMENT WASN'T WRONG in suggesting that most of us need to improve our form if we are to run like Kenenisa Bekele or reduce injuries. Trying to change how we land, however, didn't address the more important elements that create those effortless, elite movement patterns we desire.

The problem was the focus. The emphasis on foot strike put the attention on the end of the chain, rather than the beginning. Experts agree that we need to shift our focus upward to our hips, where the stride begins.

"More often than not, I see foot strike as simply being the end result of so many other things that are happening further up the kinetic chain," says David McHenry, DPT, physical therapist and strength coach for Nike's Oregon Project. "The foot is really just the end of a big kinetic whip—the leg. Core and hips are where every runner should be starting if they are really concerned with optimizing their form, maximizing their speed, and minimizing injury potential."

German sport scientist Markus Blomqvist, who has done

extensive video analysis and coaching of runners' form, says, "It's hard to tell how someone is running just by looking at the foot. You need to see the whole body. I would never just tell a runner to increase steps per minute or to land on a different part of the foot. I always include the whole body from the beginning, starting from the hips."

Brian Fullem, DPM, author of *The Runner's Guide to Healthy Feet and Ankles,* says that most running issues he encounters stem from the hips. "As a podiatrist, I get better control from the hip than I do from the foot the majority of time. What happens up above is as important or more important."

Shoes and feet have often gotten the blame for most leg injuries. Fullem points, however, to a study published in 2000 by Michael Fredericson, MD, at Stanford University, which showed that runners who suffered from iliotibial (IT) band syndrome tended to have weaker hips and that strengthening their hips allowed most to return to normal training. Other studies, including a 2011 systematic review of research in *Sports Health*, have linked weak hips to patellofemoral joint pain, commonly known as "runner's knee," and show correlations between weak hips and other injuries like shin splints and plantar fasciitis.

Beyond injury prevention, experts agree that improving your hip strength and range of motion will help you run more effectively. "That's the key," Blomqvist says. "Running with good posture and hip extension. Then everything would fall into place. The consequence of this body posture is that running is going to be much, much easier."

Jay Dicharry of the REP Biomechanics Lab in Oregon says, "You're going to have runners who run on everything from rearfoot to midfoot to forefoot, [with] forward lean and backward lean. There is no one magic angle, no one magic thing." What does make a difference? "If you can keep your posture in check and keep your hip drive up, you're going to run really, really well," he says.

"Ultimately that is what every elite athlete is working on, having more flexibility in their hips so that the foot can stay longer on the ground and pull back further and stronger," says Grant Robison, who was once an elite-level runner himself. "To a large extent, what makes an elite athlete elite is the ability to open one's hips up and create power like that."

In sum, it seems, as oft is said about pennies and dollars: Mind your hips and your feet will take care of themselves.

SIMULTANEOUS STEPS

The next four chapters will lay out tasks necessary to reclaim the stride we had before our lifestyles compromised it. The overriding goal is to get taller, more balanced, and more connected while moving our stride from in front of us to behind us so it can efficiently and powerfully push us along. The steps to achieving this include:

- Finding a new balance over our feet
- Rotating our hips back to neutral
- Stretching our shortened hip flexors
- Activating and strengthening our glutes
- Bringing our shoulders and arms back to neutral

The steps are presented sequentially, but they can and should happen simultaneously. We can't rotate our hips or hold the position very long if our hip flexors are too tight. We can't activate our glutes if our hips are forwardly rotated. We can't get our balance right if our arms are stuck in front of us. As we work on all of them, however, everything will come together, and each will make the others easier and more intuitive.

These steps form the core of this book's recommendations—you can't skip them or pick and choose one or two that you like. So, by all means, take the assessments and start work on each element as you come to it, then come back after you've finished the book and start putting the elements together.

BALANCING ACT

What is it that we want our hips to do? Many of us have never really paid much attention to them, having thought about running as starting with the legs.

The hips are the center of our body, connecting our torso to our legs. Our torso balances on our hips, and the hips are the fulcrum of the leg levers that drive the body forward. If they are not working properly, the legs are unable to provide optimal power and speed. And many of us have trouble using them properly, resulting in all sorts of inefficiencies. The most common is overstriding: reaching forward and landing in front of our torso at an angle that makes us brake with each stride and puts large stresses on our legs.

We don't overstride, however, simply because we have worn overbuilt shoes and have learned poor running habits. We do it because our lifestyles outside of running create inflexibilities, weaknesses, and poor balance, which are then reinforced while running, such that now many of us are physically incapable of striding out naturally, with our legs pushing out behind us rather than reaching in front and pulling.

Bobby McGee, who led South African Josia Thugwane to gold in the 1996 Olympic Marathon, says the goal is to get back to how we moved as 9- or 10-year-olds, before environmental circumstances changed our patterns. Over time, our ability to move has been compromised, leading to the disuse and atrophy of key muscles.

Just heading to the gym to attack these weaknesses often doesn't correct them, however. Strengthening exercises will do little good without changing how we move and recruit our muscles. "Research has shown that strengthening alone—without retraining movement patterns—does not alter mechanics," says

Harvard biomechanics researcher Irene Davis, PhD, professor at Harvard Medical School and director of the Spaulding National Running Center. "The individual must own the new pattern, or it will not be durable."

Before we can own it, we need to feel it.

Pelvic Proprioception

The key to effective hips starts with balance. Are you balanced over your feet and legs so that you are not using muscular effort to keep upright? If you can start in a neutral position, movement is a matter of smoothly shifting balance and pushing in the direction you want to go.

Balance starts with proper posture, the experts say. Proper posture is what makes some athletes look graceful and light on their feet, balanced and agile, the upper body moving effortlessly above the legs. McGee calls it "getting connected." Gerard "G.P." Pearlberg, author and online running coach, calls it "running tall" and describes it in terms such as "the jockey must sit atop the horse."

Whatever we call it, learning it takes more than trying not to slouch or sucking in our guts. Good posture is not the stilted, rigid position we adopted when our mothers yelled, "Sit up straight!" The word *posture* feels old-fashioned or military. Most of us cannot imagine maintaining such a pose for long just sitting or standing, let alone running. From an early age, we learn to dismiss calls for better posture.

To get away from old ideas of posture, it might help to think of it instead as *hip proprioception,* a fancy term that Trent Nessler, DPT, physical therapist and CEO of Accelerated Conditioning and Learning, a provider of research-based sport performance programs, uses to describe our awareness of what is going on with our hips. This includes both the position of the bones and the activation of the muscles firing around them.

Dicharry's book, *Anatomy for Runners,* centers around this concept. "It comes down to awareness and *feel*," Dicharry writes, noting that people who have habitually poor posture "don't respond to cues like *run tall* and *keep your spine in neutral.* They pretty much have no idea they have a spine, or a hip, or any muscles that control them at all."

If we are in this situation, where do we begin to learn pelvic proprioception? The first test, recommended by a wide variety of coaches and therapists, is vertical compression. Before you go any farther in this book, do it now.

VERTICAL COMPRESSION TEST

While standing, have someone behind you put his hands on your shoulders and push straight down, steadily and firmly. If your body buckles at the back and hips, you know your hips and balance are off. "If you fail that test, we don't do anything else," Dicharry says. "You're grounded until you fix that."

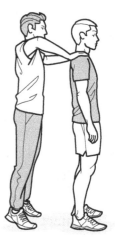

FINDING NEUTRAL

Fixing your posture is fairly simple. You can quickly improve by getting your hips stacked up correctly. To find this new, balanced posture, start by standing comfortably with your feet shoulder . Lift your arms and reach up as high as you can, as if something off a high shelf just above your fingertips— g onto your tiptoes. Without changing your hip and back position, slowly lower your arms back to your sides.

Now look down at your feet. You should be able to see the top of your shoelaces where you tie them. If not, still keeping your hips and chest tall, bring your torso forward slightly so you can see the front of your ankles, noticing how the weight shifts off your heel toward the ball of your foot.

Some people find it easier to start with this adjustment rather than reaching. While standing, place one hand on your belly button and one on your sternum. Without moving the belly-button hand, bring your sternum forward until you feel your weight balanced over your hips and equally distributed between your forefoot and heel.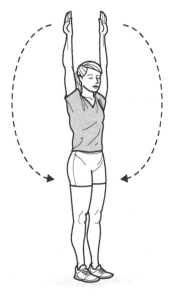

When you get into this new, tall balance, have someone push down on your shoulders again: You should now be able to withstand considerable force without strong muscular resistance.

The Tipping Point

In adjusting your posture to achieve a balanced state, you likely noted your pelvis position shifted. If you think of your pelvis as a bowl, hinged at the hip bones and controlled by the muscles in front or in back, your goal is to keep the bowl neutral and not "spill" either way. Most of us spill out the front, for reasons we'll see in the next chapter.

Danny Dreyer, author of *Chi Running,* says his tai chi teacher used this analogy in instructing him how to keep from spilling his chi energy. But you needn't buy into Eastern mysticism to benefit from this image: Dicharry and McGee also talk about not spilling cereal out of your pelvic "bowl" or water from your pelvic "bucket."

This image helps you see how to keep the pelvis aligned so you can ride better above it. The desired feeling is to have the hips "stacked under the torso"—the term McHenry uses to describe the goal of his work with elite runners. When you are able to keep the bowl from spilling, even while working hard on a run, you begin to feel the connected power as your leg drive pushes your body forward, rather than twisting your hips forward and losing its energy in the torquing.

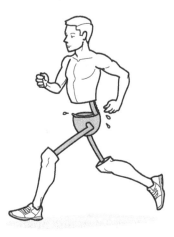

MIRROR, MIRROR

One simple way to note and feel this hip rotation is to look at it. Stand sideways in front of a full-length mirror wearing just your running shorts. Stand with your normal posture and note the angle of your waistband. By rotating your hips, try to move the band up in front. Don't worry about making the line exactly straight across—a neutral posture is not always level, and the way your shorts lie is far from precise. The point is to learn how to rotate your hips, using your lower abs to pull up in front and your glutes, or butt muscles, to pull down in back.

Be careful not to lean backward in order to change the angle of your hips. Changing the angle should, instead, reduce the curve in your lower back. This will make you taller; you will feel your chest rising and your shoulders coming up. In the end you should feel like you did after reaching for the sky, only this time you worked it up from the bottom step-by-step, rather than pulling it out straight from the top.

Now that you've rotated your hips into a neutral posture, feel your balance points: Get forward on your feet so your weight is evenly distributed on your forefeet and heels. Try to relax without dropping your hips back into the old position.

Playing with Balance

At first, assuming a neutral position may feel like you are pitching forward. In other cultures, times, and places, humans participated in daily, constant standing, walking, reaching, and carrying—which required us to maintain a balanced, strong, muscle-supported posture. Because our lifestyle doesn't require this now, many of us have gotten used to a "locked back" posture of being on our heels, with our hips tilted forward and a large arch in our spine. We are not used to having weight on our forefeet.

Because of this altered perception, we have to work on retraining our normal posture. Hang out in your neutral, balanced position and note how agile you feel. A tall, athletic posture should not feel forced—you shouldn't have to stay immobile or stiff to hold it. Rock your hips left and right, back and forth. Balance on one leg, then the other.

Rotate your hips in a wide circle, keeping your torso balanced over your hips and moving from your ankles. Bring your chest up and back, then bend and arch forward, playing with the extremes before finding a neutral, balanced middle ground. Rotate your pelvis so it goes up and down in front, exaggerating the motion, then find the middle ground that feels comfortable and balanced.

THE ELUSIVE ELITE LEAN

Once you learn to balance—with your pelvis neutral so it isn't spilling in either direction, your body comfortably resting over your hips, and your hips over your full feet—you can play with creating what McGee calls "dynamic balance." McGee points out that if you are balanced correctly during a run, you should have to move your body back into a static balance not to fall on your face when you decelerate to stop.

This is the forward lean that you see in elite runners and that is often mentioned as an element of an effective stride. Learning it, however, is so hard to get right that I, and others, are reluctant to use the word "lean." Tell someone to lean and the tendency is to drop forward at the waist, which puts you out of the balance you're working to achieve and makes everything harder and less effective.

To achieve a dynamic balance, start by getting into neutral balance, then lean forward so all of your weight is on the balls of your feet and your toes. Feel the force needed by your toes to stay upright, then lean a bit farther so that you need to take a step to keep from falling. That "just-about-to-fall" feeling is your running posture.

Robison says to focus on subtly moving your weight from your ankles. Some coaches talk about picturing yourself like a ski jumper, with your body straight from heel to head as you lean slightly forward. Be careful in particular to keep your hips forward, with no break in your straight line. Kinesiologist Ryan Green cues this by thinking when running, "Face forward—like kissing your grandmother."

In a recent *Runner's World* blog, 1968 Boston Marathon champion and longtime *Runner's World* editor Amby Burfoot discussed two recent studies, one from the University of Salford in the United Kingdom and another from the American College of Sports Medicine in Boston. "They favor a slight forward lean," Burfoot wrote. "A very, very slight lean of 3 to 4 degrees—one that's probably not detectable as you run." This is important because, as Burfoot notes, "Both studies also warn against tilting too far forward, which will almost certainly make you less efficient." It's all about balance.

"The key to the lean is that it is really subtle," says Robison. "It's a slight shift of your weight at the ankle, so your center of gravity is forward, rather than backwards."

Robison warns, "It's really hard to tell if you're leaning when you're running." As a check while on the run, he recommends getting tall, then shifting your weight backward. "You quickly feel how inefficient that is," he says. "Then slowly shift your weight over the top of your ankles again. Play with your center of gravity until you feel where it is comfortable, where it is helping you."

From Balance to Balance

When in doubt, upright is better than hunched. Work on being tall and balanced first. As you gain in proprioception, you will begin to feel the tipping point and can use it to your advantage.

Every time you move, get tall, find your neutral balance over your whole foot, then lean past that point and take the step to catch yourself. Shift your torso over that leg, staying tall, and feel yourself reach a neutral balance point over that leg. Work from this to taking multiple steps, feeling how you roll smoothly from balance to balance, gently pushing over from one to another.

Start every run this way, getting into a tall, static balance, then falling into motion, rather than reaching out with a leg and pulling yourself into motion. Feel your feet pushing off behind you and landing beneath you with a quick cadence, flicked along by your hips.

As you work on increasing your flexibility and strength, you'll be better able to keep this posture and balanced state all the time. "You as an athlete need to know neutral posture when you're standing there talking to me, need to know what it is like during an easy run, know what it is like during a long run, during speed work," Dicharry says.

But the first step is to feel it, understand it, and work to make it your comfortable default.

"How you stand is how you'll land," says Laura Bergmann, a national-class triathlete, coach, and sports rehab specialist at Evolution Performance and Rehabilitation center in Winchester, Virginia. You can't expect to maintain a new posture and balance point on the run if you don't learn it and make it a habit during the rest of your day.

GETTING MOBILE

Finding your balance is one thing, but maintaining it is another. "Some people have a problem finding it, [getting] the awareness," says Dicharry. "Some can find it but can't maintain it for more than a minute." We need to build postural endurance.

It's not just a matter of focus or strength, however. Many of us can't hold ourselves tall because it takes too much effort to rotate into neutral. The next step, therefore, has to be to improve our mobility.

4
THE PERILS OF SITTING

HOW TO RECLAIM YOUR FULL, POWERFUL STRIDE

THINK ABOUT YOUR LAST 24 hours. How many of them were spent in a sitting position? Most of us sit at work all day. We sit in the car, bus, or train on our commutes. We sit for meals. We sit all evening in front of the TV or computer. Unlike people in many cultures throughout the non-Western world, we sit instead of squat when we defecate. Many people even assume a "sitting" position on their side while sleeping. Even if we have a job now where we often stand and move, most of us sat for hours in school during our formative years. We have been sitting so long that we forget what being straight feels like.

Sitting, for the majority of our days, is one unfortunate consequence of our 21st-century lives. And sitting puts our hips in a flexed position, with our legs angled at 90 degrees or less from the front of the body.

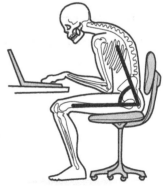

Hip flexion is not, in itself,

bad: The running motion uses hip flexion for knee lift as our legs drive forward. Effective running, however, also requires hip extension—the movement of the leg behind the torso. Good hip extension allows the leg to push backward without rotating the pelvis side to side or tipping it and torquing the back.

Watch a video of Kenenisa Bekele or other world-class runners again, focusing on their hips and thigh movement. See their thighs move far backward with each stride, their legs at the back of the stride forming a straight line from heel to shoulder. Hip extension creates the beautiful stride of the tall, powerful runner. More important than how it appears, it allows the powerful glute muscles to fully engage, pulling your thigh and knee backward while your hips stay stable, transferring power directly to forward motion. The faster we want to run, the more important this becomes.

Before we can get there, however, we need to make sure our bodies are still capable of this movement. Physical therapists, biomechanists, coaches, and elite athletes all agree that the one thing virtually every runner can benefit from is improved hip extension.

Before we go further, employ this simple test to assess your hip extension.

HIP EXTENSION TEST

Stand in front of a doorway or straight-backed chair with your back against the right side of the doorjamb and your left leg in the 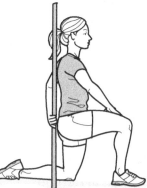 opening. Kneel down in te position with your left knee on the floor inside of the doorjamb and your right foot in front of you with your knee above it. Your left thigh should be vertical beside the doorjamb, with your back resting against the front of the doorjamb. In this position, you'll naturally have a bit of space between your lower back and the wall. Tilt your pelvis backward so the hollow between your lower back and the doorjamb disappears. Your pelvis should rotate up in front and down in back.

If you have trouble completing this rotation or feel tightness in the front of your hip and down the front of the thigh, your hip flexors are too tight. You are not alone.

HIP INFLEXIBILITY: AN EPIDEMIC FOR 21ST-CENTURY RUNNERS

Physical therapist Jay Dicharry says that at least 85 percent of runners have tight hip flexors—the muscles on the front of the leg that limit hip extension. On his short list of abilities you need in order to run effectively, number one is "enough motion to get the leg behind your body."

He has lots of company in identifying this key issue. "We *always* include exercises to improve hip extension range of motion and glute strength," says elite strength coach David McHenry.

"Hip extension is probably *the* most critical factor in effective running," says sports movement expert Brad Cox of Acumobility. T. J. Murphy, runner and coauthor (with Dr. Kelly Starrett) of the 2014 book *Ready to Run,* says that if he had to choose one mobility exercise, it would be a hip extension stretch.

Asked what every runner can do to be better, Andrew Kastor,

coach of the Mammoth Track Club, Olympian Deena Kastor (his wife), and other elites, says, "The first thing that comes to mind is hip flexor tightness and quad tightness."

Kastor tells of how, after the 2000 Sydney Olympics where Deena hobbled around the track during the 10,000-meter race with double Achilles tendinitis, he promised that it would never happen to her again. "I went to massage therapy school. I studied what the Kenyans were doing, what the Europeans were doing," Kastor says. "I'd take notes at major championships. I'd see what their physios were doing."

After all this research, Kastor reports, "The biggest thing we did to correct her Achilles problem was to stretch the shit out of her hip flexors. We just really cranked on the hip flexors."

Sitting Down on the Job

These tight hip flexors are one of the primary results of all of our sitting. At worst, the muscles on the front of our hips shorten so much that we cannot physically pull our legs backward. Unable to move our legs back, we have no choice but to reach out front and pull them back to a vertical position with each stride. The result is that we end up maintaining a "sitting" posture even when upright and running.

This causes all kinds of problems, not the least being increased loading on the knees, which often results in pain and injury—the ubiquitous "runner's knee"—as well as shin splints. Reaching results in braking with each footfall and using muscles to pull yourself along, when pushing is more effective and efficient. But trying to land beneath your body, without addressing the hip inflexibility that is keeping the leg from swinging backward, is like trying to open a door against the hinges. You either have to swing it forward to create movement, or you have to break the doorjamb to open it the other way.

That is similar to what happens in the body, with the pelvis acting like the doorjamb. Trying to extend the hip and drive the leg back without adequate hip flexor flexibility causes us to rotate the pelvis unnaturally forward, the forward "spilling" posture described in the previous chapter, which then overflexes the muscles attached at the back. Essentially, the cords on the front of the pelvis that are supposed to stretch don't, so the whole support structure has to rotate in order to allow the leg to move backward.

One of the dastardly side effects of this overrotation is that it locks out the glutes, the big muscles of the butt that are attached to the hip. With lengthened end points, the glutes are elongated and rarely engage. On many runners, the glutes have turned off and are "functionally asleep," says therapist Phil Wharton.

Disengaging the glutes robs us of power and also shifts the work to other areas not as well suited to take on the extra load: hamstrings, calves, and Achilles tendons. Experts agree that the combination of tight hips and weak glutes causes most of the common runner's pains, from shin splints to Achilles tendinitis to plantar fasciitis.

Hamstrings get the worst end of this deal, explains coach Bobby McGee. They first have to do more work than intended if the glutes are slumbering—their main task is to decelerate the shin and pull the leg down after it swings forward, not to drive the leg backward. When the hip is rotated forward from tight hip flexors, however, they also have to work in an extended, stretched position. McGee credits tight hips as causing the preponderance of hamstring soreness and injury among runners.

Loading the Rubber Bands

In addition to all the problems they cause elsewhere, overly tight hip flexors lose some of their own effectiveness as well. When they move normally, the flexors lengthen and stretch as the leg moves backward, then recoil, using their elastic energy to initially drive the forward motion of the leg. But if the hip doesn't rotate back, the flexors don't stretch, and they have to tighten an already shortened muscle to pull the knee up.

"If you achieve extension by pouring the bucket out the front, then you are not elastically loading the hip flexors," says McGee. "You have very little chance of pulling the leg through elastically—you are going to have to drag the leg through with the hip flexors."

Andrew Kastor describes how this worked for Deena after she did the work to improve her hip extension. "Opening up the hip flexors allowed her foot to travel backward in extension and also enabled the flexors to contract properly," Kastor says. "Her knee drive was coming back around because her hip flexors were no longer tight and short—she could actually use them to lift."

The Corrections

How do we correct for all of that sitting? We can try to stand more, and we should. But that works only in a few times and locations. Standing is culturally inappropriate during much of our lives. In some settings, such as in school, it isn't allowed. In others, like a work meeting, standing makes others so uncomfortable it derails social interaction and job function. Even if we started standing all the time, the majority of us have sat for so long that we need some corrective work to get the desired range of motion.

"Most runners have other jobs," says physical therapist Abby Douek, acknowledging the necessity of sitting most of the day. Douek schedules 3 or 4 days a week for work to counteract the effects of those jobs and patterns. "You cannot be a successful runner without functional training," she says.

What does that work look like? Douek assigns multiple specific exercises for her clients based on her evaluation. Lacking such an evaluation, we can choose from the many different exercises and stretches that effectively open the hips. All can work.

"There is really no magic in any one hip flexor stretch or one collection of glute-strengthening exercises versus another. The magic is simply in the consistency in doing those things," says McHenry. "Progress in these areas is made from consistency and progressive adaptation. You can't stretch your hip flexors every once in a while and do some glute-strengthening stuff on occasion and really expect any significant change to occur."

Remember what the cowboy Curly said about urban tensions in the 1991 Billy Crystal movie, *City Slickers*: "You spend 50 weeks a year getting knots in your rope and you think 2 weeks up here will untie them for you." It's the same with flexibility. We spend 167 hours a week getting our hips flexors tight and short, then we think 5 minutes will loosen and lengthen them for us.

If you're serious about improving your stride, here's where you start.

Static Stretches

The first solution for overtight hip flexors is to do something we've been told not to do any more: a long, static stretch. Numerous studies, such as those cited in an overview of research in the March 2013 *Scandinavian Journal of Medicine and Science in Sports*, have shown that static stretching before running reduces strength and power. In response, most runners have converted to dynamic warmups and active isolated (or AI) stretching.

In a situation, however, of limited mobility from shortened, overtight tissue, static stretching is one of the only ways to lengthen and release the tissue. "Improvements in flexibility come from long duration stretches that physically tear the tissue surrounding muscle fibers to increase mobility within the muscle," Dicharry explains. To avoid the negative effects, reserve static stretching for after a run, later in the day, or during a day off from running.

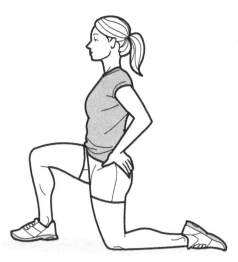

KNEELING HIP FLEXOR STRETCH

The most basic hip extension stretch doubles as a cue for posture and muscle recruitment. Done right, it isolates and focuses the stretch on the hip flexor and cues the opposing glute so that you feel the desired rotation and muscle activation. *Note:* This stretch requires keen attention to muscles and joint movements to be effective. As with all other exercises and stretches, mindless repetition will do little. If you don't feel the stretch, either adjust the way you are doing it or try a different exercise such as one described later in this chapter until you do feel it.

- **TO DO THE STRETCH:** Kneel in a lunge position with one thigh vertical over the kneeling knee and the other leg making a 90-degree angle with the knee over your front foot. Rotate your pelvis backward—imagine an axle sticking straight out of your hip bone and rotate your hip around it, so that the front comes up and the back goes down. You should feel the stretch in the muscles at the front of your hip over your kneeling leg.

- One cue that some find helpful is to place your hand on the outside of your hip with your thumb on the top front bony ridge of your pelvis and your fingers on your glute. Pull back on your thumb and, as you rotate the hip, feel the contraction of your glute in the back. Others use two hands, one "pulling" up on the front of the hip, the other on the top of the buttocks cueing downward and feeling the glute activation. Cox points out that it is the activation of the glute that causes the stretch.

- Once you are in position, you can raise the arm on your kneeling side straight up over your head and stretch upward. This will help keep the hip in the "neutral," upward-rotated position.

- Dicharry suggests doing this in a doorjamb or against a straight chair to ensure that your knee, hip, and shoulders are in a vertical line. The doorway or chair also helps you to see and cue that the arch in your back is flattening as you rotate your hip down in back and up in front.

- Hold the stretch for 3 to 5 minutes, focusing to maintain the posture and keep feeling the stretch as your hip opens. If you have trouble maintaining focus for that long, hold for 20 to 30 seconds and try alternating with one of the following stretches, like the kneeling couch stretch or the lunging lizard.

Dicharry says you need to do the stretch 4 to 6 days a week for 10 to 12 weeks to achieve the desired result. Yes, it takes that long to lengthen tissue. It is worth it. After 2 or 3 months of regular stretching, if you no longer feel tightness in the front of your hip when you get in the stretch position—tall, hip rotated, and back straight—you can stop the static, muscle-lengthening stretches and focus on dynamic mobility of the region, checking periodically for renewed tightness.

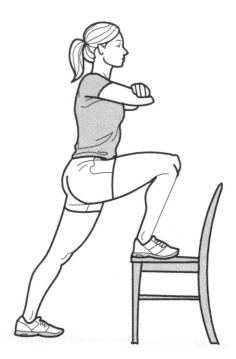

STANDING HIP STRETCH

Another simple way to stretch the hip flexor is a standing hip stretch.

- **TO DO THE STRETCH:** Stand approximately 2 feet away from a stable chair, facing it. Step up with one foot and place it on the seat. Keeping your back leg straight and torso tall so there is a straight line from your ankle to your shoulder, tighten the glute on the straight leg and lean forward with your full body, leading from the waist, until you feel a stretch in the front of the hip. Hold for 3 to 5 minutes. If you can't hold for that long, do 6 to 10 sets of 30 to 60 seconds each. This is a great stretch to do in the office. You can do it while on a phone call, for example, or when watching a video on your computer.

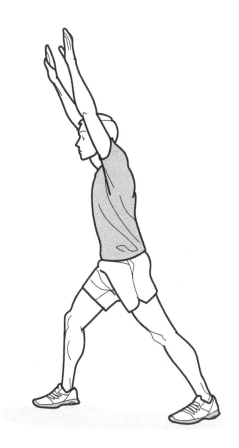

RUNNING WARRIOR

Andrew Kastor has the runners of the Mammoth Track Club do what he calls the Running Warrior Pose, an adaptation of a yoga stance.

- **TO DO THE STRETCH:** Step into a shallow lunge, then raise your arms in the air, creating a straight line from your rear heel to your hands. Contract your glute on the back leg and rotate the front of your hip upward as you stretch your torso longer. Hold for 30 seconds. When you release, drive your back foot backward with your glute before swinging it forward to the front and landing in the opposite leg position to repeat with the second leg. Repeat 5 to 10 times.

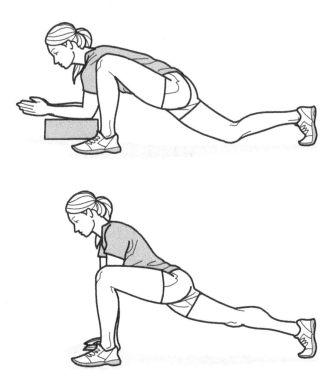

LUNGING LIZARD

This move, inspired by yoga, can provide a strong hip flexor stretch while also strengthening the glute and stretching the hamstring and other hip muscles and tendons on the other side of the body.

- **TO DO THE STRETCH:** Start by stepping forward with your left leg and dropping down into a forward lunge so the left knee is over the foot and the back knee is just touching the ground. Lower your torso inside the left leg so that your left elbow is near your left ankle. Go as far as is comfortable—midshin or all the way to resting your elbows on the ground. Keep your shoulders straight so your elbows are at a similar height with each other. You may want a pad or box under your elbows for support.

- Stretch the right hip flexor by pushing your hips forward. Enhance the stretch by squeezing your right glute to raise your right knee off the ground, forming a straight line from heel to shoulder, and stretching the front of your extended right hip. Hold for 30 to 45 seconds. Raise your torso and step through to the other leg to repeat.

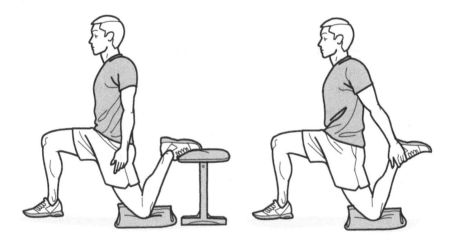

COUCH STRETCH

In his 2014 book with Murphy, *Ready to Run*, Starrett describes this stretch as a "weapons-grade technique to open up the hip." The stretch is similar to the kneeling hip flexor stretch on page 42, but adds more quad stretch by pulling up on the back leg. Starrett uses a support like a wall or a couch to hold up the back leg.

- **TO DO THE STRETCH:** Get into the stretch by first, on hands and knees, backing up to the support until one knee and lower leg (pointing upward) are touching the support. Bring the other leg forward so that the knee is over the foot and you are in a kneeling lunge pose.

- Contracting the glute on the leg propped behind you, drive the front of your hip forward and downward. Hold for 60 seconds or more. Enhance the stretch by lifting your torso while keeping your glute engaged and the line from knee to shoulder straight and tall.

- If you are flexible and coordinated enough, you can accomplish a similar stretch by assuming the kneeling hip flexor stretch and then reaching back, grabbing your back ankle, and pulling it up, stretching the quad on the front of that leg. Make sure you get your torso back into a straight, upright posture to continue the stretch on the front of the hip. From this posture, you can increase the stretch on the hip by moving it forward, or increase the stretch on the quad by pulling harder on the back leg.

THE BRETTZEL

Physical therapist and author Gray Cook has devised an excellent advanced combination stretch, which targets mobility along the front side of both the lower and upper body. It's best demonstrated in video. Google "Brettzel" to find video descriptions by Cook and Brett Jones, whom it was named after.

Dynamic Pre- or Postrun Stretches

These stretches won't physically lengthen tight tissue, but they work to relax and lubricate tissues, allowing you to access all the mobility you currently have. Since they are active and of short duration, you can use them as warmup or cooldown activities without the side effects of reduced muscle reaction and power that come with static stretches.

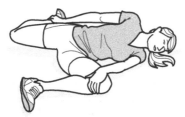

ACTIVE ISOLATED QUAD STRETCH

Active isolated (AI) stretching, popularized by physical therapists Jim and Phil Wharton, stretches by activating muscles opposite to the target muscles. This isolates the target muscle and allows it to relax while strengthening the opposing muscle in a natural coordinated effort.

The "active" part of AI stretching stems from the theory that if a muscle is stretched too far, too fast, or for too long, it protects itself with a reflexive recoil in an attempt to prevent the muscle from tearing. This occurs about 3 seconds into a stretch.

Therefore, AI stretch practitioners stretch to their natural range of motion, before the reflex kicks in, hold briefly, and then return to the start position and repeat multiple times. By using this active, repetitive motion, the muscles gain a greater range of motion over the course of each set of stretching without the muscle-damaging effect of static stretching. Kastor instructs his runners to try to increase their range of motion by an additional 1 percent with each rep.

- **TO DO THE STRETCH:** To stretch the hip flexor and quad, lie on your side with your knees curled up against your chest (in a fetal position). Slide your bottom arm under the thigh of your bottom leg and place your hand around the outside of your foot. If you can't reach the whole way, you can grasp your knee, or use a looped rope or strap.
- Reach down with your upper hand and grasp the shin, ankle, or forefoot of your upper leg. Keep your knee bent and your leg parallel to the surface you're lying on. Contract your hamstring and glutes to move the upper leg back as far as you can, using your hand to give a gentle assist at the end of the stretch. Make sure your hips stay stacked on top of each other and don't "fall open" so you are stretching the inside of the groin rather than the front of the hip. Think about pushing the top hip forward while you keep your upper leg low and behind you as you draw it back.
- Pulling the back foot closer to the butt will increase the stretch on the quadriceps. Relaxing the bend of the knee and pulling the upper leg farther back will focus the stretch on the hip flexor. Work both as you repeat the stretch 10 to 15 times, holding for less than 2 seconds each time.

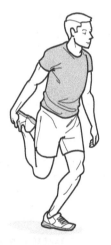

SINGLE-LEG SQUAT WITH STRETCH

An advanced move that combines strengthening with stretching is a one-leg squat with quad/hip flexor stretch. This puts you in a more dynamic position, closer to running, than the typical standing quad stretch does.

- **TO DO THE STRETCH:** Start by standing tall, raising your arms as high as you can, and stretching out your torso so your hips rotate upward in front. Lower your arms while keeping your body in the same position. Look down at your feet and bring your waist backward far enough so you can see the tops of your shoelaces. You should now be balanced over your feet with your weight evenly distributed between the heel and the ball of your feet.

- Reach down with one hand and grab your right ankle. While pulling your right knee backward, lower your body into a squat over the left leg, making sure that your left knee doesn't go forward farther than your toes. Lower yourself as far as you can, feeling the strain in your left glute and the stretch in your right front hip. You may need a wall or chair within reach to provide quick stability, but try to maintain balance over the supporting foot. Come directly back up. Repeat 10 times on each side. Work up to three sets.

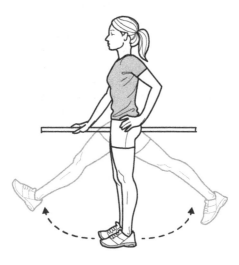

LEG SWING

An easy, dynamic way to work on hip extension is to do a linear leg swing. This is a nice warmup move, as it avoids the negative side effects of static stretching and will prime you to improve performance. It also feels good at the end of a strength-and-stretching routine to relax tissues that have been worked over hard.

- **TO DO THE LEG SWING:** Standing next to a wall, fence, or other support, first get tall by reaching up as high as you can without going on your tiptoes. Drop your arms but keep your hips and torso in the "tall" position. Swing one leg forward and back without arching your back, rotating your hips, or tipping your torso. Focus on the back swing, contracting your glute and feeling the stretch on the front of the hip. You can bend your swinging leg slightly, but don't stop the thigh as you swing your lower leg up at the end. Use the weight of your lower leg to pull the upper leg farther back. Repeat 10 times with each leg.

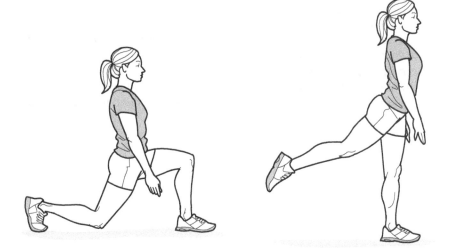

FORWARD LUNGE

Another dynamic move that mobilizes the hip flexor and many other muscles is a walking lunge.

- **TO DO THE LUNGE:** Step forward with your left foot, far enough so that your left knee is over your left foot and your right knee drops close to the ground. Keep your torso tall and your hips square to the front. Contract your right glute and drive the right hip forward. Hold for 1 to 2 seconds, then either step back and repeat 5 to 10 times with each leg, or step through with the right leg and walk forward 5 to 10 steps with each leg.

- To add to the range of motion and work your glutes at the same time, push back on the back foot after the stretch and pull it up, kicking back and upward with your full leg as you step through to a lunge on the other side.

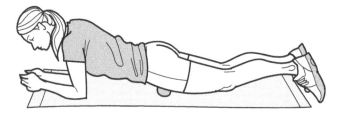

SELF-MASSAGE

A final step in mobility is to break up restrictions. Dicharry, Cox, Douek, and Starrett all recommend using a foam roller or some sort of ball—lacrosse ball, tennis ball, trigger point ball, Acumobility's stable ball—to roll out your hip flexor muscles.

- **TO DO THE MASSAGE:** Place the ball or edge of the foam roller under the front of your hip, lying prone over it. Roll from the abdomen to the top of your quad, working both up and down and left and right, teasing out and mobilizing any tender and tight spots.

WHAT ABOUT OTHER MUSCLE GROUPS?

This book is focused specifically on the muscles and connective tissues that are negatively affected by our lifestyles and that tend to compromise our running strides. The stretches and exercises outlined and illustrated here will help push you back toward your natural movements, but they are not meant to be exhaustive. You still need to be aware of other muscles that require special attention—stretching and rolling and strengthening—based on your personal patterns, weaknesses, and training.

If you are having persistent problems in an area—foot, Achilles tendon, knee, hip, back—I recommend seeing a physical therapist, even if you aren't technically injured. Many sports-med specialists offer a "prehab" assessment, where they can pinpoint areas of concern and recommend targeted interventions for you, specifically and personally.

5
REAR ENGINE

THE BEAUTY OF YOUR BACKSIDE AND HOW TO BUILD ITS STRENGTH

TO HAVE A HIP DRIVE like the elites requires not only mobility, but also strong, active glutes. The glutes are the cluster of muscles that make up your rear, the largest being the well-known gluteus maximus, or "glute max," with smaller stabilizing muscles on the sides.

Experts agree that glutes are the most powerful, efficient movers for running, and failing to use them creates serious problems. Trent Nessler, DPT, says runners' greatest strength deficiency is that they suffer from flat butts. Jordan Metzl, MD, a sports medicine physician at the Hospital for Special Surgery in New York, agrees. Metzl, a 33-time marathoner and the author of a book on running health, says, "A strong butt is the key to a happy life."

"There are a bunch of important muscles," physical therapist Jay Dicharry says. "But if you're going to spend time improving something, improve your hip extension by improving your glute max." Strengthening your glute max, he says, improves postural awareness, reduces postural fatigue, and helps reduce rotation of the leg. "The glute is super strong, has a great leverage, and [is] not going to fatigue as much as other muscles," Dicharry says. "Yeah, I want to tap into that guy—let's tap into a fatigue-resistant muscle, a muscle that creates more force."

Not only do we need strong glutes, but they need to be working. Once again, sitting for so much of the time and having permanently rotated hips has messed up our normal posture and muscle use. Our bodies have a remarkable capacity of recruiting other muscles to do the work of ones that are weak or locked out by inflexibilities. These neural patterns can become habits and feel normal. Physical therapists report that it is not uncommon to find athletes whose bodies are finding ways to work around hibernating glutes not only when running but also when trying to do exercises to work the glutes.

German sport scientist Markus Blomqvist lists "activating the glutes" as the third key—along with hip extension and posture—to start running easier and more effectively. "If an athlete's glutes are firing and the pelvis is staying stable, then the leg will work back quicker and the upper body will stay more stacked," says McGee. "Now you're getting more bang for your buck."

Runners who have weak and inactive glutes fall into what Dicharry calls the "toilet bowl of doom—a beautifully engineered screwup of epic proportions." Posture falls apart, the stride has to move in front of the torso, and other muscles compensate until they fail.

As with balance and hip position, the first thing we need to do is to learn to feel the glutes—develop glute proprioception—and ensure that they are firing at the right time. The simplest test to assess your glute activation and strength is to do a bridge.

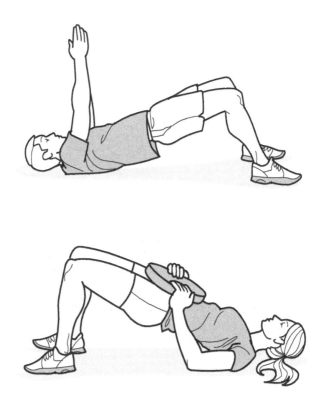

GLUTE TEST 1: THE BRIDGE

- **TO DO THE TEST:** Lie on your back with your knees up and your feet flat on the ground. Hold your arms straight out above you with palms together. Lift your hips up to make a straight bridge from shoulder to knees. Where do you feel it? If you feel stress anywhere but your butt, you aren't activating your glutes. "If you feel your back working right away, that's a huge flag," Dicharry says.

- First try changing the bridge angles to see if you can move the stress. Rock your hip angle, change your back arch, or move your feet so that you don't feel the effort in your back or your hamstrings but in the center of your butt muscles. Clench your butt and push your hips forward until you feel a stretch in the hip flexors on the front of your hip bones.

- One way to ensure that you are performing the bridge correctly is to have someone push down hard on the front of your pelvis or place a weight on the top of your pelvis. You won't be able to hold it if you aren't using your glutes. Dicharry says think about squeezing a quarter between your butt cheeks—move with your hips, not your back.

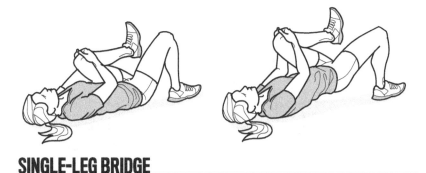

SINGLE-LEG BRIDGE

- If you have trouble isolating the glutes while in the starting bridge position, first try pulling one knee to your chest, which locks out the back's ability to arch. Then do a single-leg bridge with the other leg. The single-leg bridge also isolates one glute at a time, revealing if one is weaker or harder to activate.

Two other tests to feel your glutes activate are as follows.

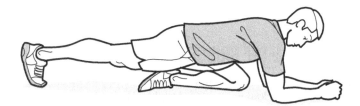

GLUTE TEST 2: PIGEON HIP EXTENSION

- **TO DO THE TEST:** Get on your hands and knees. Reach one leg straight back, then lower that knee to the ground while dropping your upper body to your elbows over the other leg tucked beneath you. Clench your butt cheeks together, then raise the back knee to straighten the leg without lifting your toes. The only muscle that can do this is the glute max. Feel it activate. Now lower the leg while keeping it contracted. This begins the work of learning to isolate the glute from surrounding muscles. Don't be discouraged if it isn't easy at first. Dicharry says people tell him "this is the hardest thing I've ever done, not from a physical aspect but mental aspect."

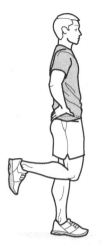

GLUTE TEST 3: STANDING HIP EXTENSION

- **TO DO THE TEST:** Stand on one leg with the other held so that the calf is parallel to the ground. Hold your hands on your hips, with your thumbs in front on your hip flexors and your fingers reaching down to feel the glutes in the dimple on the side of your butt. Drive the lifted foot backward into an imaginary wall, without allowing your pelvis to rotate forward or your spine to tip or bow. Feel your glute activate under your fingers and your hip flexor extend under your thumbs.
- Pay attention to when the glute kicks in—it should be before your hamstring on the back of your thigh tightens. Podiatrist and biomechanist Simon Bartold says mis-sequencing, with hamstring firing first, also limits your stride and stresses your hamstring. If your leg moves before the glute activates, focus on relaxing your hamstring and contracting your glute first.

OWNING IT

The task, at first, is simply to learn to feel when the glute is active and get in touch with the neural pathways in order to trigger it. After learning what it feels like for your glutes to contract, start noticing if they are working at other times.

Notice them firing when you walk: Stand tall and push your heels back, making sure your full leg, from heel to thigh, moves behind your torso, while keeping your hips squared to the front.

Actually close a door with your foot pushing behind you and feel the glute work. Lying down, roll on your stomach and raise one straight leg upward without lifting your hip, then the other.

The key time to feel if your glutes are working is, of course,

THE NEED FOR SPEED

Throughout this book, I've mostly lumped all the benefits of working on your stride together: injury prevention, ease and comfort of running, and performance enhancement. For the most part, you can do this: Counteracting the factors that compromise an effective stride will help you run better, regardless of your goal.

If your primary goal is speed, however, you likely need to focus more on the length and power of your stride than those concerned simply with ease and safety do. While many talk about "quick and short" strides, those who go fast need to have both quick and long strides. Their long strides, however, should flow out the back, not reach toward the front.

"How do you get faster?" asks Ryan Green, PhD, assistant professor of kinesiology at Southeastern Louisiana University. "Gotta drive from the glutes, the posterior. If you can teach folks how to fire from the posterior chain, that really propels them forward. Working on [the] backside makes all the difference."

The way to do this is through the same process discussed in the last three chapters: getting taller, getting your hips flexible, and building your glute power.

"It does improve performance dramatically," coach and sports rehab specialist Laura Bergmann says about the posture and flexibility work. "If you're not in a position to use your glutes, then your performance is going to suffer, because you're not using one of your most powerful muscles. I would argue that increasing your hip extension by a couple of degrees will absolutely improve your performance." She has personally seen these dramatic effects firsthand in her race times as a national-class triathlete.

If you can reduce braking by moving your stride from in front of you to behind you, you're not only going to have less risk of injury but you'll also be able to run more effectively, not sabotaging your forward progress with each step. If you can release your hip flexor, you'll be able to use less energy by not straining against it with each backward stride.

Once you've gotten your glutes to start working, if your goal is speed, you'll need to focus on building power in them. Instead of the minimum number of reps in your glute exercises, you'll want to do the max. As you when you're running. Tom Miller, PhD, exercise scientist and author of *Programmed to Run,* calls the feeling when you get it right a "glute goose" or a "hip flick" with every stride. Others call it running "from the butt."

gain in strength and coordination, you'll need to do explosive work as running fast requires power, not just strength. "Power follows strength," says coach Bobby McGee. "Power is the speed component."

"[The] research is very clear," Jay Dicharry says. "If you want to run faster, put more force in the ground." The difficulty is, it takes about half a millisecond to develop peak strength, but when running, we contact the ground for less than a half of that time. "You don't have time to develop peak strength," Dicharry says. You have to generate strength very quickly, which is where power comes in. "Strength is: Lift the TV up," Dicharry says. "Power is: Throw the TV."

Work on jump squats to build your explosive glute power. Find other plyometric-type exercises. "I think a lot of people are strong enough, but people need to work into a little bit of plyo mind-set," says McGee. He says you don't need to do full plyos, which are a quick road to injury, particularly for masters runners. "Little micro hops or step-ups—that kind of thing is very important," McGee says. "Ladder drills, quick-feet drills are essential."

After getting your stride working properly, speed, particularly in distance events, is all about the motor. You need to have an adequate aerobic engine to keep your stride going fast and long for the length of the race. And the way to build that engine is to run more. "From 95 to 98 percent of our work is running—keeping the main thing the main thing," says Andrew Kastor. Other coaches echo this, emphasizing running as the road to success.

Aerobic and muscular strength will make you faster not only by keeping your turnover and stride length going, but also by allowing you to maintain your form throughout the race. A stride that is falling apart from fatigue is less efficient. "When you let your posture compensate, you're literally working harder to run the same speed you were before your form changed," Dicharry says.

Formwork is not a magical shortcut to faster times. But focusing on it will help get you there—by making sure you're not fighting yourself with each stride, by making your runs smoother and easier, and by avoiding injury so you can be consistent and build the strength to maintain a powerful stride for the length of your runs and races.

When it clicks, you can feel the glute pulling your thigh back while your hips remain stable and connected, channeling the energy of the leg drive into forward motion. You'll start to feel the strain of hills in your butt rather than your quads. At the end of a long running week, your butt will be sorer than your thighs are. For many of us, before we get to the point where we're using our butts the way they are meant to be used during running, we have to do some supplementary work to build their strength after years of disuse.

BUILDING YOUR BUTT

If you've been running without engaging your glutes, you're going to have to strengthen them before your nervous system will trust them enough to use them again. "Most people don't use their glutes—I'm gonna make that blanket statement," says physical therapist Abby Douek. When people come to her for help, more often than not "they're going home with some butt-strengthening [exercises]."

You can strengthen your glutes with numerous exercises. The Internet is full of "build a better butt" programs. But beware: You can do a lot of these exercises and not actually recruit and work the glute. The body is clever at using the easiest route to create a movement. Also, while variety is good, too many options can raise the complexity to the point where we get overwhelmed and don't do any exercises at all or just do them mechanically, without our full focus. Better to do one or two simple things every day, or at least 3 or 4 times per week, than a bunch once a week or less often.

Here are some exercises that studies have shown to be effective and that I've found most useful and easiest to integrate into a running program.

BRIDGE

The simple bridge, described on page 55 as the first test for glute activation, doubles as a good place to start working on glute strength.

- **TO DO THE BRIDGE:** Start by finding the position where all the strain is in the center of your butt muscles and hold it for 10 seconds, then lower and repeat 3 to 5 times. Don't let your butt sag while holding. Push up until you feel the stretch in the front of the hips. Work up to holding for 30 to 45 seconds.

- As soon as you are able, add the single-leg option. Pull one leg to your chest, then bridge up with the other, keeping your hips level. Work up to 30 to 45 seconds per side, or do reps: Hold at the top for 3 to 5 seconds, lower the bridge, then repeat for 20 to 30 reps on each side.

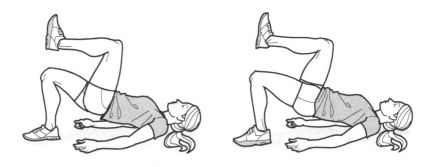

MARCHING BRIDGE

Once you can hold a bridge, you can add a "marching" option.

- **TO DO THE MARCHING BRIDGE:** While in the bridge position, raise one leg up until that foot clears the other knee. Bring the leg down and reverse, raising the opposite leg. Make sure you keep your hips level— you should be able to hold a glass of water on your belly button and not spill it. (Dicharry says to imagine it is hot chocolate or coffee and will burn you if it spills.) Start with 10 and work up to 20 to 30 steps on each side. As you fatigue, make sure your bridge doesn't sag: Concentrate on squeezing the supporting glute and pushing up at the hip.

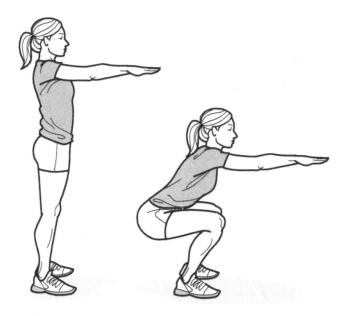

AIR SQUAT

Squats are today what crunches were in the 1990s—everybody's doing them. And for good reason: They work the glute in a powerful but simple way using your body weight, and they build a beautiful butt. Until you do them correctly, however, you won't strengthen your glutes. Instead, you will likely reinforce the movement patterns and muscle recruitment that bypass glute power.

Runners who use their quads rather than their glutes to squat most likely also swing their legs too far forward during their running stride, says Dicharry. They've learned to compensate for weak glutes and tight hip flexors by landing with their balance behind their foot, their weight supported by strong quads. For these runners, the squat, performed correctly, works not only as a strengthening tool but also as a retraining of neural pathways from a quad-dominant to a glute-dominant pattern.

- **TO DO THE SQUAT:** The key to an effective squat is to never let your knees move in front of your toes. The best way, at first, to ensure this is to put your toes under the edge of a chair with your knees lightly touching the seat (make sure you are standing tall with your balance in neutral and weight divided between the balls of your feet and your heels). Now, put your arms straight out in front of you for balance and, keeping your back straight and tall, lower into a squat.

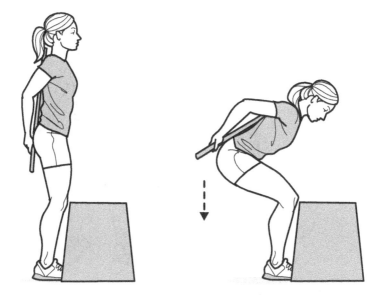

- The goal is to not push into the chair or push it forward as you drop into a squat. Lower until your thighs are parallel to the ground. To do this, you need to stick your butt far out and use your glutes to keep from falling over backward. If you do push the chair forward and lift your heels—and most people do—you have grown used to using your quads over your glutes and need to retrain your glutes and rebuild their strength. Dicharry calls this the "Chair of Death."

- To keep yourself even more in line and to make sure you aren't cheating on the balance by hunching forward, Dicharry recommends that you hold something long, like a stick, dowel, PVC pipe, or foam roller, on your back so it is touching your tailbone, the middle of your shoulders, and the back of your head. Make sure it doesn't come off of your back as you lower down.

- After working with the chair enough that you feel the balance and muscles required, you can do the squat without it. But it helps to still visually cue the posture by lining your toes up against a curb or crack in the sidewalk and watching whether your knees cross the line, making sure your heels stay on the ground.

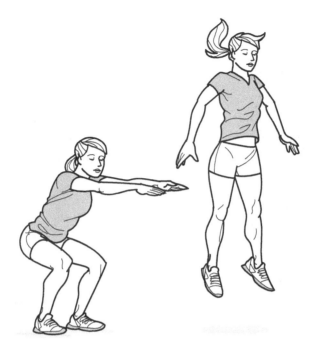

JUMP SQUAT OR ROCKET SQUAT

The final, advanced squat move is to add an explosive jump to the end of it. Jordan Metzl, MD, calls these plyometric jump squats and starts with them in his IronStrength workout series.

- **TO DO THE SQUAT:** Metzl recommends standing with your feet a bit wider than shoulder width apart and splayed slightly outward. After you lower into the squat, pushing your butt out and keeping your back straight as above, push up from your heels to explode off the floor, then land lightly and drop right back into the squat. Do 15 to start, working up to six sets of 15.

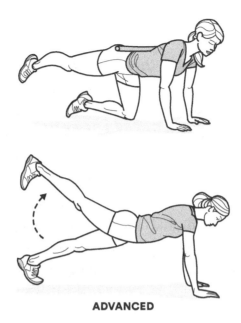

ADVANCED

BALANCED DONKEY KICK

The donkey kick uses the glute in a similar manner as running does, moving the leg back from a stable torso—but it can be difficult to perform properly to ensure that you're not compensating by rotating your back, which doesn't work the glute and instead reinforces bad muscle recruitment habits. Done right, Dicharry says, "the donkey kick is a great way to learn to keep your core in neutral while isolating the gluteus maximus to extend your hip." To accomplish this, you need to keep the kick balanced and controlled.

- **TO DO THE EXERCISE:** After getting on all fours in the "table" position with your back straight and stable, place something long, like a stick, across your lower back. Keeping your spine stable, lift one knee and extend the leg as far back as you can. Then, keeping the leg straight, lift from the butt and extend the leg slightly to the side. Keep the stick balanced and your spine level, clearly isolating the muscles in your butt and hip. Hold for 2 or 3 seconds, then lower the leg back under you and repeat with the other side. Work up to 50 reps with each leg.

- *AN ADVANCED OPTION: Once you are confident of your ability to isolate and work the glutes while keeping a neutral core, an advanced variation is to do a donkey kick from a pushup plank position. Make sure to keep the hips level and that you're feeling the work in the butt of the leg you are raising, while tightening your abdominals and holding a solid, straight line with the support leg.*

Lateral Glutes

The previous exercises mostly target the big, stride-driving glute max, but the smaller glutes, medius and minimus, are also essential to an effective stride. These muscles are often weak in runners, because of sitting and the lack of side-to-side and balancing work in the straightforward, road-running action. The glute med and min provide stability to keep the hips from dipping side to side and the knee from collapsing inward during the stride. Studies, such as ones conducted by Irene Davis's group at the University of Delaware in 2007 and 2010, have shown that weak glutes are linked to several injuries, particularly IT band syndrome and knee pain.

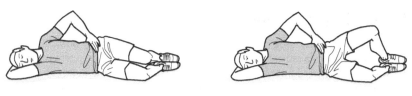

CLAMSHELL

The clamshell is an easy way to begin work on your gluteus medius.

- **TO DO THE EXERCISE:** Lie on your side with legs crooked at a 45-degree angle and your knees stacked on top of each other. Before you begin, straighten out the curve in your spine so that there is a small space between the floor and your side. This tightens your abdominals, rotates your hip up toward the front, and helps isolate the gluteus medius when you start the exercise.

- Lift your top knee as far as you can, keeping your feet together. Hold for 2 or 3 seconds and drop back to your original position. Touching the side of your butt just above and behind your hip bone, you can feel the gluteus medius activate. You can increase the intensity of this exercise by wrapping a resistance band around both legs at the top of the knee.

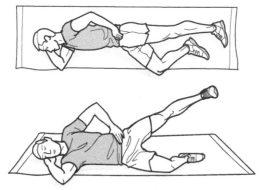

SIDE-LEG LIFT

A 2009 study from the University of North Carolina at Chapel Hill that compared numerous exercise methods showed the side-leg lift to be one of the best ways to activate and isolate the glute muscles. It is also one of the best for teaching glute activation and awareness.

- **TO DO THE LIFT:** Lying on your side, bring the knee of your lower leg up to stabilize you, then reach your upper leg out to form a straight line from your shoulder to hip. *Note:* Most runners initially do not get the top leg back and their butt forward far enough. To check, do this against a wall and make sure your shoulders, butt, and heel all touch the wall. Keep your hips stacked on top of each other and your torso forward. Bring your top shoulder forward with your arm and elbow toward the ground to help lock yourself in this position.

- Raise your top leg straight up. Hold at the top of the lift for 2 or 3 seconds, then relax and repeat 15 to 30 times with each leg.

- If you're doing this lift correctly, you will only be able to raise your leg a foot or two, reaching at most a 45-degree angle. Many people, when doing this lift, rotate their hips backward and engage the hip flexors on the front to raise their leg up past a 45-degree angle. The point isn't to raise the leg high but to contract the right muscles. To make sure you do, think about keeping the top hip directly above or a bit forward of the lower one and keeping the lifting leg straight, which, to many, feels like you are pulling it back behind you. You may need someone to stand behind you and keep a foot on the back of your butt to ensure that your body doesn't rotate and fall backward. Many runners need to work hard just to engage the right muscle to activate this lift. You can place your hand on the side of your butt just above and behind the hip bone to feel when the glute medius contracts. You should not feel the contraction on the top or front of your hip.

- *AN ADVANCED OPTION: Once you reach the top of your lift, clench the glute maximus to pull your straight, raised leg backward in the same plane, with your knee moving behind your hip. Return to the straight position and lower. Repeat 15 to 30 times with each leg.*

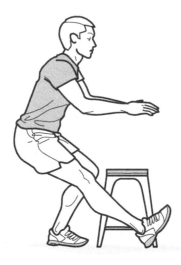

SINGLE-LEG SQUAT

The single-leg squat could be considered the graduate-level glute exercise. It doubles as a test of adequate glute strength: If you can perform it without your torso leaning over, your hip dropping to the side, or your knee diving in toward the middle, you can be confident that both your glute max and med are engaged and strong enough to keep you tall and stable during the one-leg-at-a-time action of running.

One reason not to lead with the single-leg squat is that it is easy to "cheat" here. If your balance comes forward over your toes and your knee drives out past your feet, you are using more quads than glutes and will feel the stress over your knee.

- **TO DO THE SQUAT:** To perform it correctly, you need to stick your butt out and lower it down as if you are going to sit on a chair behind you (some recommend putting a chair there to reassure you that it will catch you if you fall over backward). Make sure your supporting knee doesn't come forward farther than your toes. A chair in front of your knee can help keep you honest with this, as in the Chair of Death.

- For balance, your lifted leg should be out in front of you. You can extend your hands in front as well. Try to stand tall. Start with smaller squats: one-quarter or one-half of the way to a full-seated position where your thigh is parallel to the ground. Go deeper as you build strength and coordination. Do 5 to 10 with each leg to start, then work up to 20 reps with each leg.

WHAT ABOUT THE CORE?

Not many years ago, everyone—myself included—was focused on the core, not the hips or glutes. The answer to all life's problems was in improving your abs. Was that all wrong? Should we still worry about our core? Why are there no core exercises included here?

First, note that all the therapists, trainers, and physicians I interviewed agree the core is still important. All of the exercises and postural improvements described here and in other chapters start with engaging the core. The core provides the connection between the powerful pistons of the legs and the torso they are driving. As Dicharry says, "You can't fire a cannon from a canoe." A runner without a strong core is a canoe, unstable and easily tipped.

The difficulty is that most of the methods for working core muscles are either ineffective or counterproductive. Most already know that situps don't work the same muscles as posture exercises do: They tend to target the exterior muscles on the front of the stomach and may give you a nice-looking six-pack, but likely won't help you run better. Most of us switched to doing planks several years ago.

Dicharry says, however, that planks aren't his favorites, either. He gives two reasons: First, planks are static, holding a position for several minutes. "Running is dynamic," Dicharry says. "I'd rather people learn to feel and maintain the right muscles through movement." Second, he says many people do planks incorrectly, actually reinforcing the improper posture and imbalanced strengths they are trying to correct.

Instead, Dicharry, Douek, and others like nationally known natural running and movement expert Mark Cucuzzella, MD, recommend working the core in the context of every other movement. Engaging the core muscles is the first step, part of "getting tall" that precedes all lunges, squats, drills—and running.

First, you need to learn how to feel the muscle you want to engage. The main stabilizing muscle of the pelvis and torso is the transversus abdominis (TA), which runs along the front and side of the lower abdomen. To feel this muscle, find the top front point of your pelvis bone with your fingers. From that point, slide your fingers an inch inward toward your center line, then up an inch toward your belly button, and dig in. There are several ways to cue and identify that the right muscle is contracting—choose whichever works for you.

❭ Force a cough. This contracts the muscles quickly, but is hard to hold and replicate consciously.

❭ Push your tongue against the front of your teeth like you are saying an *S* sound with a lisp, so it almost blocks the air passage. Inhale, then push the air past your tongue in a forceful exhale. Feel how the muscles under your fingers contract. Try to make them do the same thing without blowing.

❭ Contract your abdomen as if someone were about to punch you in the belly below the waist.

Note how the contraction is low, below your navel, and deep, layered beneath the surface abs (obliques). Note also how contracting the TA complements the hip rotation you have been working on, pulling the hip up in front while the glutes pull down in back.

Once you have found the muscle, work on contracting it at will, dissociated from your breathing or other movements. Contract it for 5 to 10 seconds for several reps and work up to contracting and holding it for 30 seconds—it's longer than you think.

You can work on contracting the TA anytime—standing, sitting, or lying down. I like to do it on long, boring drives, trying to hold it for as long as I can. After reading about this core move in a 2006 *Running Times* article by physical therapist Thomas Minton, long before I focused on my running form, I started to work regularly on my TA strength and coordination. Soon, I found it greatly improved my posture and the feeling of a strong connection channeling power between my lower and upper body—particularly when I learned to keep it tight and engaged on the run.

"Activating this muscle is like kindergarten," Dicharry says. Controlling the TA and engaging the core is the prerequisite for all of the exercises recommended here.

Final note: Once you know you are working your core, you might return to doing planks. "I love planks," Douek says. "I think they are a phenomenal exercise to work multiple body parts at the same time." But, like Dicharry, she quickly adds, only "when they're done correctly—to do a plank right, you have to have a little bit of body awareness. If you are not doing it correctly, I take it out."

Here's how Douek cues a proper plank: "First thing you have to do is tuck your bottom under." By this, she means pull it down so it is in a straight line from your shoulders to your heels and rotated down in back and up in front, with your glutes and TA engaged. "Once you've tucked your bottom under, make sure your shoulder blades are pulled together. Once you've done that, make sure your bottom is still tucked under. Once you have those two pieces, drop into your heel." Do this by pushing yourself backward and downward over your feet, stretching the calf muscle.

"You need the calf length with the core tight and your shoulder blades back, in order to push off for running," Douek says.

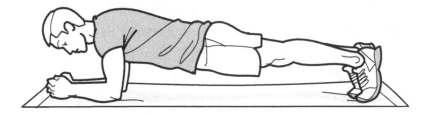

Got it? In position, you should feel the strain of holding it in your lower abdomen, connecting to your sides and shoulders and through your rotated hips (bottom tucked) to your legs, all the way to your heels. You should not be holding yourself up with your hip flexors. If you're unsure, it's best to have someone with expertise watch and cue you. From this position, and from side and back planks (where you should still have your abs tight, hips rotated, bottom tucked), you can add leg lifts to engage some of the dynamic elements of running.

6
HOW YOUR LAPTOP, SMARTPHONE, AND CAR ARE KILLING YOUR STRIDE

RESTORE YOUR NATURAL ARM SWING TO IMPROVE POSTURE AND POWER.

THE HIPS MAY BE THE body's fulcrum and its center of balance, but things that happen above the waist can, and do, also affect balance and drive. The body is all connected, all balanced on top of itself: head, shoulders, hips, knees, ankles, feet. Throw off that balance at the top, and the supporting structures need to work harder to keep the body upright, before they begin the task of pushing us forward.

Arms and hands are body parts that often show a runner's unique stride signature and ones that physical therapists and podiatrists warn about trying to change too much because arm movement can compensate for deficiencies elsewhere. A hand that kicks out to the side, for example, may be balancing a slight leg length discrepancy.

That said, we can note a few elements of effective arm posture and uses that are universal. And here, as with the hips, our lifestyles often compromise what our arms would naturally be doing if we lived as our ancestors did—using them for lifting, carrying, pushing, pulling, throwing—as well as for daily, extensive walking and running.

You don't run on your arms, but make no mistake, arms are important to running. Coaches have long maintained the importance of arms in enhancing the stride. "There is a lot more to running correctly than just getting your feet and legs working properly," wrote 1950s Olympian Gordon Pirie in his training guide, *Running Fast and Injury Free*. "What you do with your hands and arms is equally important." He devotes considerable space to describing how to hold and drive your arms—compact, vigorous, in unison with the legs in "very quick but powerful pulses."

Former elite runner Grant Robison finds it is easier for runners to focus on and change their arm rather than their leg movements. "Your arms are right by your face," Robison says. "They are easy to focus on. It really works. It is hard to think about where your foot is landing in relation to your hips. But your arms, you can make them go."

Physical therapist Abby Douek says she'll often start with the arms. "When I'm working with somebody on cues for running form, 90 percent of my form correction is arm swing."

"People think running is all about the lower body," says therapist Laura Bergmann of Evolution Performance and Rehabilitation center. "But because it is all connected, tightness up there affects down here. Tight lats and pecs, rounded shoulders, all inhibit your ability to have a tall spine when you run."

"Many problems are attributed to hips that are actually upper body mechanical problems," says mobility expert and coach Brad Cox. Cox says most everybody has some upper body problems that stem from excessive sitting and hunching.

We hunch over computers—even more now that everyone uses a laptop. We hunch over phones and video games. "Sitting is horrible," says biomechanist and marathoner Rebecca Shultz, PhD, who works as product researcher and designer for Lumo Run, a new, clip-on stride monitor. "Tech added on top is awful." And it isn't just tech; we reach forward while driving, reading, writing, eating. Everything in our lives, it seems, cues our upper body to be forward oriented.

What happens when you've spent hours, days, years in a hunched position is that you end up with inward-curved shoulders and arms that lack the ability to move backward comfortably.

"Everything we do is forward," says Bergmann. "If we look at life as a workout, we're doing a whole bunch of forward exercises, so that muscles get really short in the forward position. You try to have an arm swing, and you can't because your shoulder can't go back." So your arms end up staying in front, reaching forward or rotating and moving across the front of your body.

PUSH YOUR ARMS BACKWARD

If you look at a video of elite runners, however, you'll see that invariably, regardless of how high they carry their arms or what their arms and hands do in front of their body, they drive their elbows far back with each stride.

"A powerful arm drive is 100 percent backward," Robison says. "It's just the recoil that brings it forward. The faster and the stronger you can drive your arm back, the quicker your arm turnover will be, and the more reaction your feet will have in relation to that."

"If your arms are out in front of you, your trunk starts to bend at your waist," Douek says. "If your trunk is bent at your waist, you're sitting into your hip flexors, which means you're not using your glutes and you're going to overuse your hamstrings."

Cox names poor hip extension as the first of numerous problems created by rolled, hunched shoulders. When your upper body isn't working right, it is hard to get good hip extension both because you can't get your spine in neutral and because your balance is forward so you need to bring your leg forward to support you. Cox adds that a collapsed chest reduces your breathing capacity, and it restricts the connection between the lat muscles on the back of your shoulder and the opposite glute, which keeps the glute from firing properly. "All three things affect balance," Cox says.

In sum, tight, rotated shoulders can sabotage all the gains you might get from the posture, hip flexibility, and strength work of the previous chapters, throwing off your balance and drive.

CUE THE DRIVE

How do you know if your arms are swinging effectively? One simple cue is to pay attention to your hands. If, while looking forward at the road ahead, you can see your hands during the full stroke while you run, you're probably carrying them too far forward. They should disappear below and behind your peripheral vision on each backswing. Hands left in front not only don't cue a backward-driving leg action but instead tend to swing left and right, rotating the torso to maintain balance and diverting energy sideways that could be propelling you forward.

You can also assess effective arm swing by looking at yourself when you pass a reflective storefront window. Or have someone take a photo of you from the side as you run. Note whether you can see some air between your elbow and your back on the backswing of each arm. In his book, *Meb for Mortals*, Olympic medalist Meb Keflezighi says he looks at his shadow for the bright triangle of light between his torso and upper and lower arms.

Both Douek and Bob Glover, longtime coach for the New York Road Runners and author of the bestselling *The Runner's Handbook*, recommend a simple, tactile cue: On every stride, your hand should brush your waistband as it passes by, backward and forward. Other coaches talk about grabbing something from your hip pocket or pulling a gun from a side holster. The key is that your hand comes back to your hip or a bit farther with each stride.

Coach Bobby McGee teaches a "Velcro drill" where you imagine the insides of your wrists are stuck to your shirt at the side of your torso to keep them down and back as you start to run. As you warm up, you can relax and let your arms swing comfortably and efficiently, staying in an elbows-back position.

Use a Posture Bar

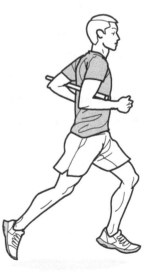

Tom Miller, PhD, exercise scientist, masters coach, and author of *Programmed to Run*, recommends carrying a 2-foot-long, ½-inch-thick PVC pipe across your back, held in the crook of each elbow, to keep your shoulders back and your arms from driving too far forward. The posture is a bit exaggerated as it doesn't let your arms swing as far forward as they usually would, but it is great for getting the feel of driving back rather than forward and mandates a shift in posture and balance—pushing your torso forward and not allowing an overstride.

Miller suggests using the pipe for the first half mile of an out-and-back run, leaving it in a secure place, then picking it up for the last half mile to reinforce the posture when you are fatigued. Or, if running in a group, pass it around on the run, using it for 3 to 5 minutes every few miles.

Try a Posture Strap

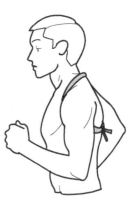

In my coaching experience, runners dislike using the bar behind their back—those who need it most dislike it passionately. Another simple solution that is less obtrusive but provides a subtle tactile cue and reminder is to use a posture strap. My runners have universally appreciated this, saying that it not only made them stand taller and swing their arms better, but opened their chest and helped their breathing.

To create a posture strap, cut a 6-inch-wide tube out of the torso of an old T-shirt. First pull it on your torso, under your armpits, then pull the front up over your head to rest on the back of your neck, with the loops pulling your shoulders back. Alternatively, you can put one arm through and tighten it across the front of the shoulder, then reach back with the other hand and loop the other end around that shoulder. Once in place, reach up behind your neck and pull it back so that the tension is greater across your back than it is on the back of your neck, which should not be pulled forward. If the band is too loose, falling down the back and not pulling back on your shoulders, tie a knot on one end of the loop to reduce its length and increase its pull.

Open Up

You may, however, need to do more than retrain your habits to get your arm to swing behind you. Many people are so hunched and rotated they can no longer get their arms in a position to allow a relaxed backward swing. In this case, forcing a backward arm drive is likely to simply cause tension and create excessive torso rotation.

"I don't think everybody needs an actual physical therapy intervention," Douek says. "But most people need foam rolling and a daily stretching routine for shoulders and back, because we are so forward as people—our shoulders are forward, our heads are forward." Cuing your shoulders back and standing tall isn't enough to correct the hunching that starts in middle school and is reinforced daily by driving and desk work. "Everybody needs some kind of routine to fix it—unless you work as a backstroke instructor," Douek says.

"Getting your elbows back is often inhibited by tight chest and shoulder muscles," says Bergmann. "The problem is, no matter how much you concentrate on it, the tissue is shortened. I can give you all the exercises in the world, but you've got to release that tissue." To correct this, you need to stretch the muscles in the front of the body—chest, sides, shoulders, and arms—and strengthen the muscles in the back.

How do you know if your shoulders are overly tight? Bergmann provides a simple test: Stand in front of a mirror with your arms relaxed at your sides. If you see the back of your hands rather than your thumb and index finger, that means your shoulders are internally rotated, turning your arms inward.

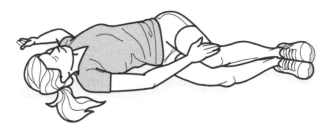

SHOULDER AND CHEST MOBILITY ASSESSMENT AND STRETCH

Cox presents a more robust test to see if you have the mobility to get your shoulders and arms back into a position to swing freely and effectively.

Start by lying on your right side with your shoulders and hips stacked on top of each other. Reach your right hand over your left knee and hold on to it to keep it in place and not let it rotate backward. Lift your left arm straight up and rotate it backward, reaching out as you drop your arm. Attempt to drop your left shoulder to the ground without rotating your hip backward.

If you can't reach the floor, you need to work on your upper body mobility. One stretch is to continue to do the evaluation, working on a greater range of motion. Cox recommends that you first inhale a deep breath into your belly as you rotate your shoulder over, then release as you lower your shoulder toward the floor. Repeat 5 times on each side.

Mobilize Your Shoulders

Stretching by itself, however, won't get you where you want to go if you have adhesions in your muscles and connective tissue restricting their movement. An overly tight chest and stretched back creates more problems than impeding effective arm movement, says Cox. He says nearly everyone needs to target mobility in the mid- to upper back and around the trunk and chest.

"This is fundamental to power transfer in the running stride," Cox says. "In many ways, more important than the shoulder itself, because you can have a mobile shoulder but no ability to transfer that power to the hips if the thoracic spine is restricted."

To work on those, you'll need some deep massage and release techniques. Not for the faint of heart, this mobilization technique will cause you to gasp in pain. But Cox says it is essential to get into the tissue and break up blockages. "Unfortunately, if you do not do something about the tissue problem, you will just create tension somewhere else," Cox says. "You can only fight [restricted tissue] for so long by consciously pulling yourself into good posture or stretching. It's going to win. That's why people are constantly fighting the same stuff every day—unless you get after that in a proactive way, it's not necessarily worth doing." Here's how you get after it.

Place two balls on the floor next to each other. Acumobility sells balls with a flat side that stay in place better, but tennis or lacrosse balls will also do well and have the added advantage of being more mobile so you can find the tight spots more easily. Lie down on your back on top of them, with your spine between them at shoulder blade level. Bridge up by tightening your glutes, so that you create a straight line from your knees to your shoulders, resting on top of the balls. Raise your arms from your sides to straight up and then over until they are touching the ground behind your head. Then rotate them outward like a snow angel. Repeat 5 to 10 times. Move the balls up or down the spine to find tender spots and repeat the arm roll 5 to 10 times at each spot.

"You get a lot of bang for your buck," Cox says about this

exercise. "In 2 minutes, even though it sucks, you can work through that."

After getting the muscles to release so that you can lower all the way to the floor on the assessment above, Cox says other stretches and exercises are adequate for releasing tension and generating bloodflow—although you should occasionally test to ensure that your day job hasn't made you hunched and tight again.

If putting your body weight on top of the massage balls is too much at first, Douek suggests a slightly less aggressive method. Standing with your back to a wall, place the balls on either side of your spine between your shoulder blades, held up with pressure between your back and the wall. Roll up and down on the balls using mini squats, applying as much pressure against the balls as you are able to tolerate.

You can also roll out your back lying atop a foam roller. This will work if you don't have any significant restrictions and is a way to keep the area mobile after you've released bound-up tissues. Resting on the foam roller, placed horizontally across your upper back, put your hands behind your head and do a slight crunch, then bridge up with your legs, applying pressure into the roller. Roll up and down your back and hit any sore spots on either side. Roll for 3 to 5 minutes.

Note: *Anyone with osteoporosis should stay clear of this move as it can apply dangerous pressure to the bones of your spine.*

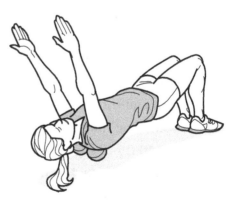

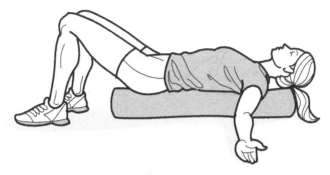

FOAM ROLLER CHEST STRETCH

This stretch, recommended by physical therapists Bergmann and Jay Dicharry, works on opening up your chest using gravity and time. When we're rotated forward, not only do the muscles on the back get overstretched and become weak but those on the front get tight and shortened. Like the hip flexors discussed earlier, it takes time to lengthen these shortened tissues, requiring long, static stretching.

- **TO DO THE STRETCH:** To stretch your chest, lie on a foam roller aligned with your spine, facing upward with your arms out to the side, palms up. Your head and tailbone should be on the roller, with your knees bent and your feet on the floor. Check that your lower back isn't excessively arched—one hand width between back and roller is okay, but two hands' width is too much. Tuck your chin down so your head and neck are aligned and straight.

- Stay in this position ideally for 10 minutes, but at least for 3 to 5 minutes, letting your shoulders pull your chest open. Then slowly stand up and do a set of 10 rows as if pulling on two vertical chest-high handles, focusing on bringing the shoulder blades back and together, as if cracking a nut between them, while keeping your shoulders low and relaxed. Do this 2 times a week and for 5 minutes before a run whenever you can.

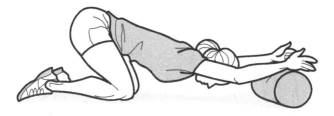

LAT STRETCH WITH ROLLER

Lying on your back on the foam roller as on page 83 is also a good position in which to assess the tightness of your lats, the large muscles alongside the back edges of your chest. In the same position as the previous stretch, simply raise your arms overhead with your palms facing each other and then lower them directly over your head until you achieve a straight line from your hips to your fingers. If you can't get to a straight line, or if you can get there only by arching your lower back up, you could use work on relaxing your lats.

Tight lats contribute to pulling the shoulders forward and limit the range of shoulder and arm movement. Like other muscles discussed here, lat tightness often stems from lifestyle issues—they get shortened when we stay hunched over and never open enough to stretch them to their full range of motion. Running from the arm to the pelvis, they not only affect shoulders and arms but simultaneously contribute to pulling the back of your pelvis up, compounding the overrotation and "spilling" out the front caused by tight hip flexors.

- **TO DO THE STRETCH:** To stretch your lats, kneel in front of a foam roller with your toes facing backward and lower yourself down so your butt is resting on your heels. Reach out in front of you with both arms resting on the foam roller, thumbs up and palms facing each other. Lower your body so that your arms are straight in line with your torso, with your head between them. Yoga calls this a "child's pose." Hold this position, ideally for 5 to 10 minutes, pushing down gently, feeling the stretch on the backs of your arms and the sides of your chest below your armpits, relaxing with deep breaths, trying to go lower with each exhale. Alternatively, you can gently roll forward and back, rocking from left to right to feel more stretch on each side.

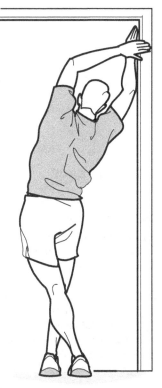

DOORWAY LAT STRETCH

One more way Douek recommends stretching your lats is by making a bow with your body in a doorway.

- **TO DO THE STRETCH:** Stand near the center of the doorway, lift your hands over your head, and get tall—engaging your core, lifting your chest, and rotating your hips down in back and up in front. Lean your body over to the right to grab the door frame. Reach your left arm over your right arm to reach up as high as you comfortably can. Then cross your right leg over your left leg so you make your body into the shape of a C or an archery bow from your left ankle to your left hand. You should feel the stretch in both of your lats—the backside of your chest below the armpits—and toward your lower back. Your body should not be rotated—make sure your pelvis is facing forward. The stretch should feel gentle, not forced. Switch to your other side, reaching toward the top left corner of the doorway with your right hand and crossing your left foot in front of your right. To lengthen the lats, hold on each side for up to 3 minutes. You can also stretch for 10- to 15-second intervals throughout the day.

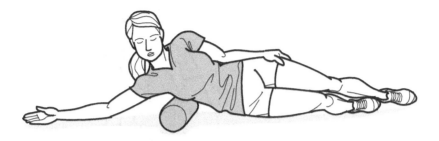

FOAM ROLLER LAT RELEASE

To further release your lats and to rub out restrictions, you can self-massage them with a foam roller.

- **TO DO THE RELEASE:** Lie on your right side with your right leg bent, supporting you, and your left leg stretched farther out, somewhat straighter. Place the roller under the side of your chest, below your armpit. Keeping your arm stretched out straight with your thumb pointed up, use your left leg to push your body up and down, rolling from your shoulder to midchest. Explore, rolling farther onto your back and farther toward your chest to find tight spots. Lift your body into a side plank to apply more pressure when you are ready. Reverse sides and repeat. This is often a painful exercise—embrace it like you would a hard interval workout, knowing that it is going to hurt, but it's so worth it.

Arm Swing Exercises

In *The Whartons' Back Book,* Jim and Phil Wharton recommend two arm swings that are effective at getting the shoulders back and cuing the muscles that will keep them there.

First is a series of open-arm swings designed to stretch the muscles in the chest and shoulders using the opposing muscles between your shoulder blades. Stand tall with your feet shoulder width apart. With your arms straight, bring your hands together in front of you at about waist height. Inhale. Contracting the muscles in the middle of your upper back so that they bring your shoulder blades together, swing your arms back as far as they can go. Exhale. Swing your arms forward and repeat, raising them slightly every time until you reach shoulder height (see opposite).

Start again at the beginning, by the waist, and work up the body a second time.

Douek recommends using gravity to work the back muscles harder by starting this exercise with your chest against a Swiss ball in a plank position, then, keeping your shoulders low, raising your arms up behind you.

Second is an arm swing that stretches the front of your upper arms and shoulders while also working the muscles on the back side, similar to the running motion. Start by standing tall with your feet shoulder width apart and your hands comfortably by your sides. Swing your arms straight back, keeping your elbows locked and your palms facing each other (see the illustration on page 88). Keep your shoulders low and relaxed. After taking a few swings to open up, touch your fingertips together at the back of the stretch or gently interlace them. Keeping your elbows locked,

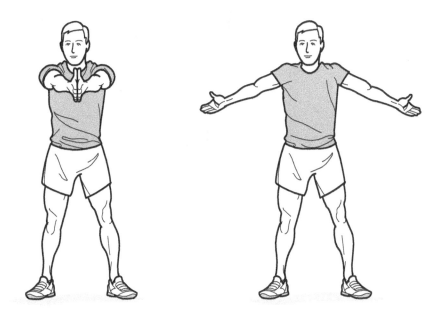

gently raise your arms slightly while pulling back and squeezing your shoulder blades together. Hold for 2 seconds and release. Do 10 reps.

You can also hold this pose with your fingers locked and your shoulders pulled back and down, to stretch and lengthen your pecs.

This exercise can also be done by lying on a Swiss ball and raising your arms behind and above you.

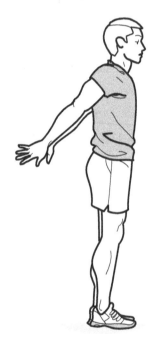

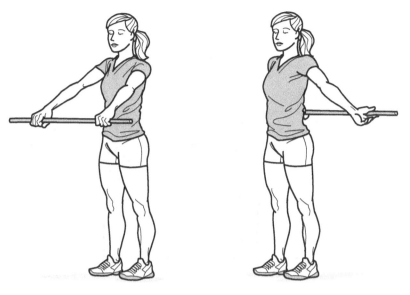

SHOULDER PASS-THROUGH

Running coach Andrew Kastor recommends doing the pass-through, an exercise popular with CrossFitters, as another method of loosening shoulders and increasing mobility.

- **TO DO THE EXERCISE:** Start by holding a bar (such as a broomstick or PVC pipe) in front of you with an overhand grip that's about 4 feet wide. Keeping your arms straight, raise the bar to an overhead position, then all the way around until the bar hits your backside. Take care to stay tall with your chest over your hips, your torso straight, and your core and glutes engaged—don't let your back arch or your hips drop forward. If you can't get all the way around, try a wider grip. Work toward a narrower grip as your shoulder flexibility increases. You can also reverse your grip, starting with an underhand grip in front, for a slightly different stretch. Do 15 to 30 reps.

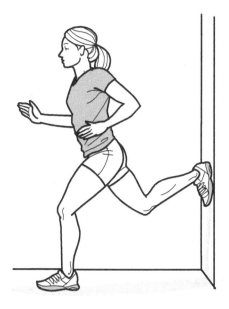

INTEGRATIVE WALL PUSH-OFF

Cox recommends a final integrative move that cues glute activation and the connection between that and arm drive.

- **TO DO THE EXERCISE:** Standing facing away from a wall, raise your right foot and place it onto the wall behind you in the running posture. Pushing against the wall, fire the glute on the right side while simultaneously driving your right arm forward and left arm back. Feel the power flowing through your connected core from the leg drive all the way to your open shoulders. Reverse with your left leg against the wall. Do 5 times on each side.

WHAT ABOUT THE HEAD?

Moving all the way to the top of the body, we come to the head. Anyone who saw the film *Jerry Maguire* knows that "the human head weighs 8 pounds." Most actually weigh about 10 to 11 pounds, which is a large load to balance atop this moving stack of body parts.

Ideally, the head should be balanced atop the shoulders, leaning neither forward nor backward nor side to side. Coach Andrew

Kastor lists having your head over your shoulders as one of his first keys to good form, the first step to getting tall and balanced. "Because when your head comes over your shoulders, it raises your center of gravity up," Kastor says, while having it tipped leads to a forward lean that stresses everything down to your toes.

Harvard professor Daniel Lieberman and biologist Dennis Bramble, in their famous *Nature* article, argue that the ability to balance the head and keep it still while the body bobs and the shoulders rotate is a unique human characteristic that allows us to run. Our bodies will keep our heads still no matter what posture we assume, but an unbalanced one will require more energy and create tensions in the supporting structures below.

Just like our arms and shoulders, we tend to tip our heads forward and down during many of our daily activities. While reading this, your head is likely tipped forward, looking down at the book. To not be, you would have to hold the book at eye level in front of your head. Try it and note what happens to your head and neck. Think about all the time you spend with your neck tipped forward: reading, on your laptop, over your smartphone.

Phil Wharton recommends standing against a wall to assess your alignment. Start by backing up to put your heels against the wall. Bend your knees a bit to unlock them, then push your butt, shoulders, and the back of your head against the wall. Try to get as tall as possible, raising your shoulders, rotating your hips back to reduce the curve of your spine. Then step away from the wall and try to relax in this posture. If you quickly adjust by bringing your head forward, you're not alone.

But this forward-head posture has a cost. In *The Physiology of the Joints, Volume 3*, orthopaedic surgeon Adalbert I. Kapandji, MD, says that for every inch the head moves forward from being balanced over the shoulders, it gains 10 pounds in terms of the force needed to be generated by the muscles to hold it up. So a head tilted 2 inches is pulling forward with 30 pounds of pressure that you need to hold up and balance with your spine, hips, and legs, exacerbating all the problems discussed above caused by rounded shoulders, such as restricted breathing and limited hip extension.

A study conducted at Gonzaga University found that changing neck posture didn't have a significant effect on runners' economy, but did strongly influence their perceived effort. So working on this may not have the priority of improving hip posture, strengths, and mobility, but will help you feel smoother and faster, as part of getting more balanced.

While improving your shoulder and hip mobility will get you more upright and balanced so that you can better feel the influence of your head, unfortunately, there are no easy corrections to a forward-tilted head except to change your postural habits. Once you've done the Wharton wall test, try to get close to this posture as much as you can during your day. Think about carrying a pail of water or balancing an egg on your head. Play with your head position, bringing it forward and back until you reach a comfortable balance while doing your one-leg balance exercises. This is particularly effective with your eyes closed, when you can feel how muscles all the way up and down the kinetic chain react to a loss of balance.

For exercises, Phil Wharton recommends putting your hands on your jawbone and gently pulling backward and tipping your head upward while contracting the muscles on the back of your neck. Repeat 5 to 10 times.

Kastor has athletes do isometric exercises for the back of their neck. To do this, while lying down on the ground, facing upward, try to push the back of your head into the ground. Hold briefly, relax, and repeat 5 to 10 times. In *Meb for Mortals,* Keflezighi recommends putting a squishy ball between your forehead and a wall and pushing against it 10 times for a couple of seconds to strengthen the muscles on the front of your neck as well.

On the run, raise your sights to the horizon—or at least a position 30 meters down the road or the runner in front of you—instead of looking at the ground right in front of your feet. Kastor tells runners to pull their chins back during the run, aligning the head over the shoulders.

Most of all, run tall. This one cue can help pull your head back up over your shoulders, as well as keep your chest up, shoulders back, and hips rotated and aligned in neutral.

7
THE BASE

STRENGTHENING THE PLATFORM YOU BALANCE ON

IF WE'RE GOING TO RUN tall and balanced, quick and light, eventually we have to focus on our feet. Previous chapters have detailed how the feet often receive inordinate attention when people think about stride. We obsess over how they land, how they move once they land, and how they are supported by the shoes beneath them. This is partially due to the promise of and hoopla over footwear, and partially because feet, at the end of the chain and in contact with the ground, are easy to observe. It is far simpler, for example, to look for heel strike versus forefoot strike than to judge hip angle, even if the foot strike doesn't tell you as much about what is happening in the stride.

Make no mistake, however—feet also receive attention because they are important. While other factors higher up the chain, in the hips, core, and arms, determine how well you balance over your feet and where your feet land relative to the body, once on the ground, your feet provide the platform on which you balance.

"Let's take a skyscraper that has 100 levels," says renowned biomechanical researcher Benno Nigg. "If you have a problem at level 25, are you going to solve it at level 50? You'd solve it at the foundation."

The task, Nigg explains, is to correct any imbalance in support as quickly as possible, using the small muscles of the feet. Those muscles are designed to react to tiny changes as your foot lands, quickly aligning the foot and forming supporting structures. "Your reaction with the small muscles is very early," Nigg says. "So the excursion before changing and controlling is much smaller. If it becomes greater, then you have to use the big muscles—then the small muscles don't work anymore."

Bottom line: If your foot doesn't react to the surface or doesn't have the strength to form the supporting arches, you'll use more energy calling on big muscles in the calf, thigh, and hips trying to stay upright and in control of your stride. And you'll do it less effectively because you're starting from an imbalanced position, and these muscles and their connecting tissues are designed for propulsive power, not for producing the stability your feet are supposed to take care of.

WEAK FOUNDATIONS

Unfortunately, as with the hips, the majority of people today do not have adequate foot strength and proprioception—the ability to sense the surface and instantly react. In this case, the blame for our weaknesses goes to shoes.

Before we go on, rest assured that I'm not going to recommend that you throw your shoes away and run barefoot. Given most of our environments and histories—with ubiquitous hard and sharp surfaces underfoot and having worn shoes virtually since birth—common sense and research say that running shoes are necessary and good. People run faster and use less energy with some sort of foot covering—even Ethiopian Abebe Bikila wore shoes for his second Olympic marathon gold in 1964. Which shoes are best, however, is specific to the individual and is the topic for another chapter. (See Chapter 11.)

In relation to foot effectiveness, experts agree that shoes create weakness. "Wearing shoes all the time compromises foot strength," says podiatrist Brian Fullem, author of *The Runner's Guide to Healthy Feet and Ankles*. "If you support it all the time, you're not using those muscles."

Fellow sports podiatrist Rob Conenello says that too many of us, from an early age, are being lured by fashion and false claims into wearing too much shoe. "One of the biggest issues I see in my patients [is that] their feet are inherently weak," Conenello says.

Physical therapist Abby Douek often sees runners who have been in a stability shoe for a long time and are clearly not meant to be. "When somebody's been in a stability shoe with a high arch, and [they] go to a neutral shoe and lose that little crutch, that's when things become problematic," she says.

We desire comfort and protection, for us and for our children, thus we buy shoes that protect and coddle. But when shoes keep our feet from acting as they are meant to, they atrophy—like an arm in a cast or a body in a La-Z-Boy does. "The muscles around the ankle should stabilize; the muscles in the foot should build the arch and shorten the plantar fascia," says Nigg. "All these things disappear [when you wear overly supportive shoes], because you don't need them anymore."

The body is very efficient; it doesn't send resources to parts that aren't calling for them.

Getting Bare

The first step in regaining foot strength is to get barefoot.

"If you're not training barefoot, which most people don't do, that is a problem," says Nigg. "Because [when you are] barefoot, you use your muscles much more. The shoe takes over certain functions that these muscles in the foot and ankle joint should do. The more shoe you build, the less you use those muscles."

Again, this doesn't mean you should throw out your shoes and head out the door barefoot. "If you like running barefoot all the time, that's fine," says Nigg. "If that is comfortable for you, no problem. Nothing wrong with that." But he and others agree that most people are more comfortable in shoes, and that is what they should wear to run.

"I don't teach barefoot running, but teach barefoot strengthening all day long," says Douek. "Barefoot, single-leg strengthening is important."

To gain foot strength and coordination, get barefoot at other times. Take off your shoes at home and walk around. You can wear socks to keep warm and still get many of the foot-strengthening benefits, but going totally bare increases how well you feel the ground and also works on toughening the skin on the bottom of your feet. Work up to being barefoot the whole time you are home. Take off your shoes when you're in your yard or in a grassy park, playing ball with your kids. Take off your shoes when you're doing dynamic stretching and running drills. Start to feel your feet as mobile, tactile, active extremities, not dumb, blunt lumps—more like your hands than your ears.

And, yes, take off your shoes and run some on a smooth, grassy ball field, golf course, park, or lawn. Do only a few easy, shuffling strides to start—you're learning new patterns and don't want to strain weak and underutilized foot muscles. Let it become comfortable, a little more at a time, until you can run the length of the field several times at a variety of paces without any duress.

While you are awakening your feet, you can start to strengthen them and build their coordination. The following exercises can be done nearly any time you can set your feet free—sitting in the evening, working at your desk, while eating breakfast—as well as at focused times before or after workouts.

As you gain foot strength, you'll find you need to spend less time on the ground and less energy balancing, both of which help you stride quicker, lighter, and easier. A 2016 study from the University of Western Australia also showed that if you allow your arch to compress fully during the stride, you gain as much as 6 percent in efficiency from the elastic recoil when it bounces back. But you need adequate foot strength to use the dynamic, springlike arch and not have it overly supported by a built-up shoe or rigid orthotic.

Foot Splay

The most basic foot-strengthening move is simply to splay your toes as wide as they can go. This not only puts your toes in their natural position, before they became cramped and squeezed by shoes, but a study has shown it also to be one of the best ways to activate the key muscle that runs from your heel to your big toe and supports the arch.

Try pulling your toes as wide apart as possible, focusing particularly on moving the big toe toward the middle of the body, away from the other toes. You will feel the arch muscles contract. Hold for 10 seconds and relax. Start with 5 repetitions and build up to 25 to 30.

Note: If you have a bunion, the ability to perform this exercise may be compromised and the short-foot exercise on page 102 will be better. However, also note that, if you have a bunion, some podiatrists, like Ray McClanahan of Portland, Oregon, don't believe it is a genetic disorder that you just have to live with but is instead a result of having your big toe turned in after years in constrictive shoes. The first step you need to take is to get your toe back into line through stretches and devices like McClanahan's Correct Toes—a plastic toe spreader.

"It is physically impossible to strengthen a muscle that is stretched beyond its proper length-to-tension relationship," McClanahan says. "Instead of debating what are the best exercises to strengthen the feet, we should be asking ourselves why feet get weak and deformed to begin with." The best path seems to be working on multiple areas: Strengthen however you can while you are straightening and improving the ability of the toe and muscles to act as they did originally. See more on this topic in Chapter 11, which focuses on footwear.

Toe Yoga

Several podiatrists and coaches recommend what natural running expert Mark Cucuzzella, MD, calls "toe yoga." Like the foot splay, this involves isolating and working the toes of the foot independently.

While sitting or standing, start by lifting the big toe without lifting the other four. If you can't do this, assist it with your hand, or place a thin book or board (clipboard, cutting board) under the big toe and pull up while you push down with your other toes. If you can't raise it to 30 degrees even with assistance, you need to work on improving the flexibility of the plantar fascia by massaging out tight spots on the bottom of your foot with your thumbs or a ball.

Second, drive the big toe into the ground while lifting the other four. Keep the ball of the foot on the ground—lifting the ball and curling your toes reveals that you are using muscles in your shin. Those muscles are important as well, but when they dominate, it's indicative of a lack of foot muscle activation and coordination, which provide the initial balance and stable stance. "About 85 percent of your foot control comes from the big toe," says Cucuzzella.

Once you can isolate the toe, practice lifting and holding it briefly, then driving it into the ground. Alternate for several minutes. You can do this most any time. "High school and college runners are sitting at a desk all the time," says Conenello. "They could just focus on pushing their big toe into the ground during a lecture." You can do the same at your desk at work, or anywhere, really. Start to notice the big toe while you are running, providing stability during your stance and power and coordination during pushoff. Think about pushing your big toe down with each step, the stride rolling over it and exploding forward as it uses the recoil power of the arch to push off.

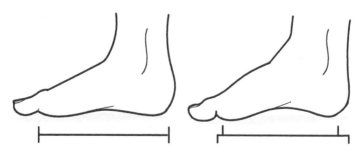

SHORT-FOOT EXERCISE OR DOMING

Developed by Czech physiologist and postural expert Vladimir Janda, MD, and recommended by many PTs and coaches, this short-foot exercise strengthens the arch and cues strong arch formation. While toe-curling exercises (opposite) work the feet muscles, they also engage global muscles farther up the leg. The short-foot exercise isolates the small, local muscles responsible for forming the arch.

One of the many benefits of strengthening your arch is to reduce stress on the bottom of your foot. "By doing doming, you're going to put a lot less stress on the fascia," says Conenello. "The plantar fascia is not a muscle, it is connective tissue. It shouldn't be acting as a support. If everything else is weak, it is going to be overutilized." Many runners, myself included, find PF pain disappears after doing regular short-foot workouts.

- **TO DO THE EXERCISE:** Start by sitting in a chair with your bare feet arranged so they are flat on the floor and comfortably beneath your knees. Without curling your toes, bring the ball of your foot closer to your heel. Your arch will dome up as your foot shortens. Initially, you may have to reach under your arch and pull up gently to cue the motion. When you reach the shortest, highest position you can, hold there and push down on your entire foot, feeling how it supports weight on a tripod formed by your heel and the ball of your foot under the big toe and the little toe. Hold for 6 seconds and relax. Repeat 5 to 10 times.

- Once you feel comfortable performing this while sitting, proceed to standing, then to standing on one leg. Advance to doing single-leg deadlifts and squats over the short foot. Do the short-foot exercise before lunges and barefoot running until it becomes second nature.

Foot/Ankle Strength and Coordination

While the intrinsic muscles in the foot are critical for support and the first line of defense against imbalance, the muscles in the ankle are just behind them in terms of their importance. They also suffer when we wear too stable, too constraining shoes and don't provide opportunity for them to work.

Nigg has been successful helping runners with ankle weakness by simply pushing their feet against a resistance in six directions: up/down, forward/back, left/right. The resistance can come from a length of rubber strength–band tubing, but it can just as well be a wall, your own legs, a leg of a chair, a table leg, or another piece of furniture. You can do this anytime and anywhere. Push as hard as you can, hold for 10 seconds, and release. Repeat 5 times.

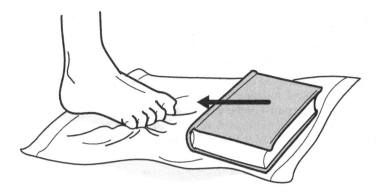

TOWEL PULL

This more structured foot/ankle exercise recommended by the Whartons, authors of *The Whartons' Complete Strength Book*, and others employs a kitchen or bath towel.

- **TO DO THE EXERCISE:** Spread a towel in front of a straight chair lengthwise, stretching straight out from the front legs. Sit on the edge of the chair so that your knees are over your ankles with your bare feet comfortably flat on the edge of the towel. Without moving your heel, contract your foot to bunch up the towel and draw it toward you. Start with the short-foot move (opposite), pulling with the ball of your foot, then contract your toes to pull farther. Continue until you run out of towel. Complete two towel lengths with each foot. As it gets easier to perform, add a weight to the end of the towel, such as a book, and gradually increase the weight over time.

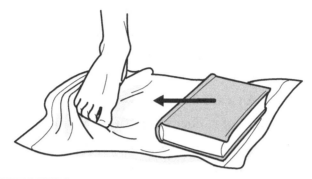

SIDEWAYS PULL

- **TO DO THE EXERCISE:** Spread a towel sideways in front of a straight chair so that the edge is in front of the chair and the length stretches out to the right side of a seated person. Sit on the edge of the chair so that your knees are over your ankles with your bare feet comfortably flat on the floor and the right foot on the edge of the towel. Without lifting your heel, grab the towel with your little toe and curl it under your foot toward your big toe, pulling the towel to the left. Keep your heel on the ground, raise your forefoot, move to the right, and repeat the sweeping motion to the left. Continue until you run out of towel. Do two towel lengths.

- Next, spread the towel to your left and put your right foot on the right edge of the towel. Keeping your heel on the floor, grab the towel with your big toe and curl it under your foot, sweeping the towel to the right. Without lifting your heel, move your forefoot back to the left and repeat the sweeping motion to the right. Continue until you run out of towel. Do two towel lengths.

- Repeat the above exercise with your left foot, pulling the towel both left and right. As these get easier to perform, add a weight to the end of the towel, such as a book, and gradually increase the weight over time.

Conenello finds it more interesting to use small objects to make it a challenge. He suggests lining up five pens or pencils on one side and using one foot to move them all to the side and back, then using the other foot. As to how you grab them, "the most important one is the great toe, because that's the one we propel off," Conenello says. "But if you can pick them up with different toes, it is better." McClanahan recommends picking up small beanbags, which allows you to utilize all of your toes in a doming action.

8
GOT RHYTHM?

THE BENEFITS—AND LIMITS— OF A FASTER ROLLING STRIDE

A FAST CADENCE HAS BEEN one of the most universally accepted and preached elements of running well. Just about every runner has been told that she turns over too slowly and should increase her cadence to be more efficient and reduce injury—and/or to be able to run in less supportive shoes. But, like foot strike, research and experts increasingly say that cadence is more personal and variable than we've been led to believe and that trying to match a prescribed rate—particularly without addressing other elements of form—can be counterproductive and even harmful.

Before we get into the excesses of high-cadence advice, let's look at why cadence is important and why it has received so much attention. Cadence, or turnover, is simply how many steps you take per minute. In general, faster runners turn over more quickly than slower runners do. That's not surprising: Speed in running is a function of stride rate and stride length. To run faster, one or the other, or both, must increase.

If, however, you maintain the same speed and change one variable, you must also vary the other—as your stride rate goes up, your stride length comes down. And playing with that ratio has been at the center of the focus on cadence, as the most common inefficiency in form is to overstride—reaching in front of the body with an exaggerated, long stride.

"Overstriding is widely accepted as poor form," says Bryan Heiderscheit, PhD, director of the Runner's Clinic at the University of Wisconsin Sports Medicine Center and a leading researcher on cadence. "But it's far easier to coach on cadence than it is to tell a runner to decrease their stride length by x centimeters."

Grant Robison, Olympian and cofounder of Good Form Run-

GETTING TIRED: FATIGUE AND FORM

It's one thing to talk about your running form when you're feeling fresh, but it's another thing altogether when you start to fall apart on a run or in a race. Our phrase "fall apart" reflects what happens under fatigue: Like a wax figure melting in the sun, you start to crumble. As your posture sags, you lose the spring in your step, your stride shortens, and your cadence lags. At the extreme, your limbs start to thrash or you descend into an ugly, barely moving survival shuffle. The ability to hold your form together through the length of a race is a large part of what makes winners.

Every element of the work described in previous chapters is important when it comes to maintaining good form. The flexibility elements let you achieve and hold your posture without fighting your own body. The neuromuscular patterning trains you to make a tall posture and quickly turn over your default pattern so you don't have to expend excessive mental energy to maintain it. Most important, however, is the strength to hold the posture, stride rate, and length throughout your run.

Former elite runner, now coach, Lee Troop says, "Things start to break away in your form during that middle third of the workout or race. A lot of it has to do with your core strength." In most areas, Troop normally recommends simply running more. But he'll give his athletes work on their abdomen and glutes to do, "so they don't slump or lose that form," he says. "The higher they sit, the better stride rate they have, and the more they can push forward, rather than [sitting] low and slumped and lose that efficiency. Especially when getting miles."

Biomechanics researcher Jay Dicharry says it all comes together—it's a

ning, says cadence is often the easiest element to think about because it doesn't require a lot of body awareness, thus making it a great place to start. "If you can find a way to improve your cadence," Robison says, "your foot strike and a lot of the efficiency stuff will come along on its own."

Besides the pragmatic aspect of cadence being an easy variable to play with, people have focused on it because changing it often works: Research shows that when runners increase their turnover, they reduce impact on their knees and hips and often improve their stride mechanics. Studies, such as 2011 research

continuum: You can't separate learning better form from having the ability to maintain it. "It's the awareness that 'here's what I'm trying to do' *and* the strength aspect," he says. "You have to do it for the full event."

To build the strength takes first activating the muscles, to make sure you're using the right ones. "You need to build postural endurance," Dicharry says. "Can you hold the position for a long time; can you maintain that?" Then you add drills, repeatedly moving in the patterns you'll use running until they become second nature. Meanwhile, you integrate those patterns more and more into your running, and you run enough to be able to hold your form for the length of your event.

There are no real shortcuts. "A lot of things take time—and come with more miles and more strength," Troop says.

One note about that time required: If you rush it and push it, you're far more likely to suffer an injury. If you can't maintain your form throughout your miles, you are not only putting the stress of the activity on your body, but adding the stress of doing it poorly, using your muscles and joints in inefficient ways. This is the experience of many marathoners. As distance runners we pride ourselves on pushing through, using mind over matter, but if we are repeatedly running past our ability to run well, we are reinforcing poor habits and setting ourselves up for failure.

You can run longer and easier than you can imagine now. But to get there requires focused work and incremental improvements over time, not sporadic, Herculean efforts that leave you broken.

by Heiderscheit, have shown that runners with a lower cadence have a higher risk of developing injuries such as shin splints. Another study, conducted in 2015 at the University of Massachusetts, Amherst, found that after increasing stride rate, runners had a less pronounced heel strike and reduced inward turning of the thigh, which is tied to injuries like iliotibial band (ITB) syndrome and knee pain.

Those who turn over faster spend less time in the air, thus tending to bounce less, and they take shorter strides, which tends to reduce the braking that occurs when you land with your foot far in front of your body. "Increasing turnover will help your chances of your foot landing closer to or underneath your pelvis, reducing overstriding tendencies, and increase your lower extremity stiffness with less bounce and braking in your steps," says Heiderscheit. In sum, taking more steps often helps people run smoother and lighter.

THE MAGICAL 180

There's also no doubt that elite runners turn their feet over fast. That observation is, in fact, where the focus on cadence started. In his book, *Daniels' Running Formula,* Jack Daniels, PhD, reported that runners in the 1984 Olympic games, both male and female, from the 1500 meter to the marathon, all (but one) ran at 180 steps per minute or faster. That number has stuck as the ideal, with conventional wisdom stating that elites keep this cadence even when running at slow paces—and so should every other runner.

That oversimplification is where the ubiquitous advice about high-cadence running falls down. "The idea that there is a single optimum for all flies in the face of the science," says Heiderscheit, who has conducted much of the research showing the benefits of high cadence. "We always gravitate toward a simple rule. We've oversimplified this. The 180 from the Olympic observations of Jack Daniels—it wasn't that 180 resulted in this great performance, [it was that] runners just didn't get below 180. Of course, these were elite runners and runners who were racing at very high speeds—much different than your recreational, novice runners."

"There is no single effective cadence for everyone," Dicharry writes in *Anatomy for Runners*. "Differences in genetics and training impact individual elasticity and likely account for a lot of the variability. . . . Research shows that both too long and too short of a stance time increases muscle work." The emphasis on high cadence comes when performance is the only goal. "If you are a highly competitive runner at the national and international level, it makes sense to utilize higher cadence as a tool to improve performance."

Coaches' advice reflects this. Bobby McGee has his world-class athletes aim to be above 180, even when running very slowly. He looks for three ranges: "Easy stuff, 188 to 192. Racing at 192 to 198. Striding, faster stuff, 220." But most of us never reach the speeds that require such a fast rhythm.

The nonelite masses of runners need a different range. After working with thousands of runners through his Good Form Running clinics, Robison says, "There will be outliers—you're going to have extremes on either ends—but for most people, you're going to have a range. If you drop your cadence below 160, you're outside the zone of efficiency, or if you try to force it and go 194, you're working way harder than you need to at a certain pace. While there isn't a magic number, there is an efficient range and you won't see a lot outside of it."

McGee also gives 160 as the lowest rate the average male runner wants to be turning over (he thinks women should be slightly faster). "If you're running much lower than 160 steps a minute, you're actually not running," McGee says. "You're doing a little plyometric hop from one leg to the other."

Heiderscheit agrees that there is a lower limit, but given his experience with less-than-elite runners, finds this "hopping" in runners who are doing 135 to 145 steps per minute. It's hard to give a lowest appropriate number given variations in pace and mechanics.

Heiderscheit is flexible with the optimal rate as well, while agreeing on the general range. "Not that 180 isn't a good, general target," he says. "But I'm completely comfortable many times with 170—quite a few people even in the upper 160s. I don't see 180 as being this absolute or absolute minimum."

A recent study by Heiderscheit and colleagues showed that high school runners with slower cadence had a higher incidence of shin injuries. The dividing line, however, was below 168 and above 172. So "170 is the new 180," quips biomechanist and marathoner Rebecca Shultz of Lumo Bodytech. Based on new research, Lumo recently revised their advice on cadence so that it is linked to the user's pace, with a different goal for those running 10-minute miles than for those running faster.

That allowance reflects another concession form experts are acknowledging: that runners use different cadences for different speeds. Contrary to the conventional wisdom, Heiderscheit maintains, "Obviously, step rate changes with speed—it is highly, highly associated with speed." Even elites, while having a faster cadence in general, vary with speed.

An example: One day I was running beside 2:14 marathoner Max King, and he assured me that he ran around 175-plus strides per minute even going easy. I clocked him at 8:00/mile and he was turning over at 166, whereupon he conceded that he had never been measured running slower than about 6:30/mile. That is much slower than his race paces, but hardly "easy" for most runners. So you shouldn't be alarmed if your cadence is 10 steps per minute slower at a 9:00/mile pace than it is at a 6:30/mile pace.

Heiderscheit also says that individuals differ. "It is so much a function of where they are starting and what you are seeing with their mechanics overall," says Heiderscheit. Which means you shouldn't compare your cadence with your training partner's, either.

I experienced a glaring personal example of the one exception to the "one-size-fits-all" cadence rule last fall, when I had the privilege of running with Martin Grüning, longtime editor of *Runner's World*, Germany. Grüning isn't a slow, recreational athlete but an accomplished, lifetime runner; he once ran 2:13 for the marathon and still, at age 53, posted a 2:44 last year.

We went out for a morning run at about a 7:30 pace. Running beside him, I felt like the Road Runner, with my legs spinning under me while he loped along. While I tend to turn over in the low 170s per minute range (and am always thinking I need to speed up), his stride rate was obviously much lower than the supposed 180 ideal. He said he's never paid any attention to it and that no one had ever analyzed his stride. In fact, he found my observation rather amusing.

Later, I asked him if he would measure his cadence with a Garmin: He reported a stride rate of 159 steps/minute at a comfortable 7:40/mile pace—a full 20 steps/minute slower than many recommend, just outside the threshold of "acceptable," according to most experts.

Grüning's stride works, however. Not only is he fast, but he's been resilient and relatively injury-free. He pushes off powerfully, with a high knee drive and long air time, but doesn't overstride or brake excessively. He has no reason to try to alter his cadence, nor does he have any intention of doing so.

DANGERS OF SPEEDY STRIDES

Several experts say that while he is an outlier with a particularly low cadence, runners like Grüning, who fall below prescribed rates, may be better off not trying to increase their cadence. Physical therapist Abby Douek has measured hundreds of runners' strides in the past year using a video gait analysis system. She has seen a far wider variety in effective cadences than expected. Before recommending someone change, she first examines other elements of his stride.

"If his ground contact time and body flight time are a great ratio, I don't want necessarily to mess with that because he is being very efficient with how his feet are hitting the ground," Douek says. "If we start turning him over too quickly, is he going to stop using his glutes, going to be more vertical, start spinning his hamstrings, make his calves too tight?"

Others agree that a faster cadence doesn't always produce the desired results. While Harvard professor Irene Davis names "relatively high cadence" as one of the first elements of good form, she also says, "It should be noted that a high cadence, alone, does not guarantee a low rate of loading [high impact scores]. We have seen numerous runners with high cadences *and* rear foot strike and excessively high rates of loading."

Heiderscheit says, "The generic 'just increase your step rate,' doesn't work universally. There are people who can increase their step rate and get this really wonky form. They way overuse their hip flexors, and their performance is just in the toilet." You've no doubt seen this form in runners—a prancing, quick, and, yes, often light landing, but all in the front of their body, reaching forward and pulling themselves along a tiny patch of the road with each step.

Excessive turnover causes runners to pick up their feet too quickly. "The biggest thing, when you do increase too much, [is that] you start to lose your stride to the back," Douek says. "With too rapid of a turnover, you get out of your glutes and into your hamstring. You get a high kick to the back instead of an extended leg. That is the biggest danger you'll see."

In the past decade, as minimalism and good form advice pushed high cadence, Douek has seen a rash of runners who mindlessly increased their turnover. "Everybody said, have a high cadence [and] you'll get midfoot stance," Douek says. "And that probably is true, but there was no regard whatsoever to what happened from midfoot to full-leg extension, [what happens during] pushoff. It's the midfoot stance to toe off that has been disregarded with the talk about cadence. That's the part of the stride that needs to be worked on the most, and that's the part of the stride that may slow cadence down."

And it's not just performance that suffered. "When somebody does increase their cadence too much, I've got hamstring injuries in my office," Douek says.

YOUR UNIQUE RHYTHM

If 180 isn't a magic number, and you can get in trouble by excessively increasing your cadence, should you even concern yourself with your turnover? As with all of life, it depends.

Research dating from the early 1980s shows that, as in other aspects of form, experienced runners tend to naturally select a preferred rate of turnover that optimizes their oxygen uptake. In other words, your preferred cadence is the one that feels the easiest to you. Increasing your turnover is going to increase your metabolic cost: You're going to need more energy to run. So, in terms of efficiency, there is no reason to change.

That said, studies, such as a longitudinal observation of distance runners at Penn State in the late 1970s, have also shown that as runners get more experienced and better trained, their turnover increases and gets closer to its optimal efficiency. Heiderscheit sees this happen with runners he observes in his University of Wisconsin clinic. "When people are new to running, they run with a lower cadence; as they gain more experience, it naturally increases," he says.

This illustrates the point that optimization occurs for the body you have at this moment: If you have restrictions or weaknesses, your body will optimize around them. You can't say "that's the way I am" until you've assessed and improved every variable as much as possible.

PREREQUISITES

This chapter is placed here, two-thirds of the way through the book, for a reason. While cadence is important, increasingly it seems similar to foot strike in that it is more of a consequence of other factors than a driver. Trying to improve cadence without addressing the issues discussed previously is what can get runners in trouble. To borrow the financial adage again, "Mind your hips, and your cadence (as well as your foot strike) will take care of itself."

If you have gotten this far without addressing posture, hip flexibility, glute strength, and upper body mobility, go back and pay attention to them. You won't do yourself any favors trying to turn over faster without first addressing those elements.

"You can't even think about cadence until you have fixed those other things," says Douek. "Until you have the strength to push off, if you don't have the flexibility to extend that leg to the back, then as soon as you start to increase your cadence, you're going to sit right into your hamstrings and hip flexors."

Even if you don't develop injuries or make your stride even more ineffective, it is nearly impossible to improve your cadence much without first changing your dynamics. You have to work on cadence in conjunction with improving your balance and hip drive, because you simply won't be able to turn over quickly and comfortably when you are reaching and pulling through each stride. Instead, you'll end up working far harder and soon fall back to a slower rate.

"If you're going to increase your step rate, also try to land with your foot closer under your hips," Heiderscheit says. "You don't want to keep reaching in front of yourself." My experience as a runner and coach confirms this: A faster cadence comes, in fact, as you learn to run tall, land closer, and push back—all part of the same process.

"Other things need to happen before this happens," Douek says. "Once you've done these things, the cadence almost would have happened already."

WHY CHANGE?

Accepting that cadence must be part of a larger process of improving your mechanics, it remains, however, something easy to focus on and measure. And there are reasons you may want to consciously increase it, even if it means creating more work for your "engine" of lungs, heart, and circulatory system.

Avoid Injury

The primary reason people advise a faster cadence is to help cure or prevent injury. If you suffer from recurring or chronic pain in your knees, hips, Achilles, or feet, running with a higher cadence may help you by reducing the strain—because it will help you reduce overstriding, which puts strain on your legs and contributes to your slower cadence. Yes, it's a circle.

"From an injury standpoint, there seems to be a shift," says Heiderscheit. "People who are running at a slightly low cadence can reduce impact by increasing [their cadence]."

He doesn't assign a target rate, but goes by trial and error, or more accurately, trial and relief. "If there is a certain pain associated with running, whatever your turnover is, measure it at a particular speed," he recommends. "Then go for a trial run with an increase of 5 to 8 percent, and see if it changes your symptoms. If it does, great, use that strategy for a period of time to get those symptoms under control."

While the new rhythm may reduce stress, it still may require more energy, and you need not stay there forever. "That doesn't mean it becomes your new preferred pattern," Heiderscheit says. You may find, however, that you adapt and the new rhythm becomes your new preferred one.

Vary Your Patterns

The second reason to play with cadence stems from that last observation: Changing your cadence can shake things up and create new patterns. The important first step is to ensure that you have the mobility and strength to stride effectively. But that is not enough. As we'll discuss more in the next chapter, changing patterns requires more than changing the parameters of your stride.

Your movement patterns are firmly entrenched by years of habit, so before your body can consider doing something new, you have to give it a chance to feel the new possibilities by forcing or tricking it into new movement patterns. Cadence, being easy to manipulate and easy to measure, is a great way to vary your stride after you've improved some of your capabilities, particularly because, if implemented correctly, it can help correct inefficiencies caused by overstriding.

While he agrees that pushing for 180 was an arbitrary target of their Good Form Running program that may have been too fast or too slow for some, Robison maintains, "I think cadence is probably the biggest tool for somebody to use to work on their stride, because it does use other parts of your brain and body than straight up trying to figure out where your hips are or whatever. You can just focus on a beep [from a metronome] or a rhythm, and it is a different part of your brain."

The focus on holding a cadence and the ways it makes you alter your mechanics to achieve a new rhythm make it effective for challenging your awareness and starting the work of rewiring your neuromuscular patterns. "If you increase your cadence, it is going to affect what is going on with a lot of your body," Robison says. "I think there is definitely a range to it, but it is one of the best tools for wrapping your brain around [stride change] and seeing a difference, without diving in too deep."

It may feel weird, it may feel harder—but that is partially the point. As you focus your attention in order to keep your stride rate up, you start to note how your legs are moving, where your feet are landing, where your balance falls. In working to make the new cadence feel less weird, you start to create new movement patterns. As you continue to hold a faster rate, your body begins to make itself efficient, moving toward a more effective stride.

Assess Your Progress

Monitoring and experimenting with a new cadence is also a way to assess your progress in changing your stride patterns. The goal is to run tall, keep your hips rotated so everything is stacked and connected, open your hip flexors to produce more hip extension behind you, and keep your chest open and arms driving backward. Barring the possibility of having someone videotape you regularly, none of those things is easy to observe (and even a video can be relatively hard to interpret).

But cadence is simple and quickly observable, even on the run, with new wearable devices and smartwatches. If we see cadence as the result rather than the goal, we're less likely to fall into the errors of excessive turnover, and we can use it as a way to monitor progress as we seek to change from reaching to pushing and to run lighter and smoother.

In my experience, I often start a run, and if I get tired, I can fall into an old pattern of sitting back and pulling through. If I don't notice this pattern through body proprioception—my hamstrings pulling a bit when driving my knee forward, or a feeling of hitting harder on my heels—I'll glance at my Garmin and see a low cadence. I can change it instantly, by getting taller, getting my arms back and chest forward, spending less time on the ground, and turning over quicker—all one process, all connected—and suddenly I'm dancing along lightly again. My cadence then goes up, giving me feedback that the form change is working, without focusing on the cadence as the goal.

Perform Better

In a similar fashion, cadence is one of the first noticeable manifestations that form is starting to fall apart due to fatigue. McGee says that consistent cadence is one of the best indicators of racing effectiveness. "If, when racing a 10K, you're losing that cadence throughout the run, then we have some fatigue and it is showing up in your cadence," he says. "Runners at the end of a race will have various cadences; pay attention to the one that is starting to lose cadence—that's the one who is going to pop pretty soon."

It happens on less-arduous runs, too, as you lose focus and the readily available energy to stride quickly. Your body, sensing aerobic fatigue, searches for the most economical way to continue to propel itself and thus lowers the cadence. While it may take more aerobic energy, keeping the cadence high is an effective "mind over matter" training technique that spares muscles and joints from undue stress and prepares you for faster running.

When considering performance and cadence, we get into a chicken-or-egg conundrum. It is not certain whether the preferred movement pattern is the most economical because your body has optimized your physical parameters or if it is most economical because you have become accustomed to that pattern and your muscles and nervous system are trained and familiar with that movement. It is likely some of both. But since better-trained, more advanced athletes almost always prefer a faster cadence, it seems to be worthwhile to attempt to train ourselves to turn over faster and see if our bodies will adapt.

Observing our culture and lifestyles, there appear to be reasons why we might fall into slower-than-optimal cadences. A personal theory that experts find plausible is that we rarely, if ever, learned to run for transportation. I've watched kids in Kenya heading to school carrying backpacks, and they naturally fall into small, quick strides that carry them faster than a walk but do not require much power to sustain. When they want to go fast, they continue this fast turnover and extend their stride and flight time.

In contrast, after their preschool age of innocence, kids' introduction to running in the United States is often tied closely to team sports where the emphasis is speed and power, and they walk when they have any distance to cover on foot. So they learn to take big strides to run with power, and when they go long, they continue to take big strides, but fall into walking-type patterns. McGee has observed that runners who come from power sports tend to keep a "lumbering stride." And Heiderscheit agrees that walking muscle patterns spill over to running.

"If you look at the mechanics of an overstrider, it is akin to walking," Heiderscheit says. "What we see with a lot of novice runners, the motor pattern of walking is still pretty dominant. When walking, to go faster, you land farther ahead—you land on your heel. A lot of runners utilize those more dominant strategies of walking."

That preferred pattern can and does change, however. "Over time, as they begin to understand running more and the mechanics of it, you see this higher turnover start to emerge," Heiderscheit says. Whatever the reason for the initial pattern, it seems reasonable that, in conjunction with improving mechanics, speeding up your step rate is progress toward becoming a more advanced runner for most.

In the end, if your goal is to go fast, you'll want to do both: turn over fast and have a long, powerful stride. Taking a shorter stride and turning over faster won't initially make you speedier. But practicing a faster cadence and shorter stride, in conjunction with mobility and strength work, can make the mechanics and neurological pathways of a faster turnover smoother. Once learned, at a slower pace, you will be able to keep your stride going faster, for longer, when you speed up by lengthening your stride with powerful pushoffs.

HOW TO STEP FASTER

Increasing your cadence is as simple as trying to take quicker steps. To quantify your cadence, you can count steps against a clock, but many GPS watches now will give you cadence in real time, while clip-on wearables measure it and display it on a mobile phone app or Web site after the run.

If you're using a watch or an app in real time, you can see changes as you make them. If you're counting or looking at a postrun measurement, you can cue a faster cadence matching your steps to the ticks of a metronome, which you can find as a free app on your phone or in an inexpensive clip-on beeper.

As you start to increase cadence, Robison says to be careful that you don't just run harder with the same long overstride. He has runners start by jogging in place at a higher than normal cadence, then speed up slowly while maintaining the same cadence. Natural running expert Mark Cucuzzella, MD, leads people through a similar process barefoot, to help cue the soft, close-to-the-body landing desired.

One way to practice your new balance is to run close to the front of a treadmill, so you can't reach out forward, while maintaining pace and stride rate. Or you can run close behind a baby stroller, if you're fortunate enough to have a little one to run with.

Other cues can help. "Some runners have difficulty changing their turnover by counting steps," says Heiderscheit. "They start to swing their arms into rhythm and then everything falls into place. [They use] their arm swing as the entry to make the changes in their gait rather than going to the feet."

The 1950s Olympian Gordon Pirie advocated consciously stopping the forward motion of the arms to cue a quicker stride. "Try to take a quicker stride than is natural. Quicken up! Get your feet back onto the ground as quickly as possible," he wrote in *Running Fast and Injury Free.* "This can be achieved by strong arm stopping, which causes the foot to land quickly but lightly on the ball/front of the foot. Do not wait for the leg and foot to drift away and land on its own out in front whenever it wants. Make it snappy and quick."

McGee ties the improvement to your posture. To get faster, he advises runners to shift their balance forward, as we discussed in Chapter 3. "Drop the chest just a little, get nice and stacked," McGee says. "Immediately their cadence will go up. Don't hold yourself in [an] upright, overly safety-seeking position."

This connection between lean and cadence becomes very apparent if you try running on a motorless treadmill like the TrueForm Runner. You have to lean and shift your balance to get moving, but lean too far and you'll quickly be sprinting to keep up. As discussed earlier, be careful that any lean is full body, from the ankle, not from being bent at the waist.

The beeping of a metronome or constantly checking your watch can get old quickly. Check early to set a rhythm, and then you can come back to it periodically. As you become more competent at holding the turnover, check your stride rate later in a run when you become fatigued to ensure you don't fall back into a slower cadence.

Are You Striding Too Quickly?

Whatever your reason, all of the experts I spoke to agreed that you should increase your cadence gradually. Add 5 percent to start and play around at that rate until it becomes comfortable and sustainable before you add more. When do you stop increasing? If we've thrown out 180 as the goal, how do you know when you're going fast enough?

Heiderscheit says, "I don't have a good strategy yet. It would be nice to say, 'measure x for 5 minutes and you'll have a good answer.'"

For experienced runners who know their bodies well, he says perceived effort is a good strategy. "That is pretty strongly correlated with a lot of oxygen use measures. You don't need to go with heart rate or being hooked up in a lab." While recognizing that neurological pathways and muscle memory need to be rewired to new patterns, you've probably reached the limit of what works for you when a faster cadence starts to require increasingly more effort.

You also have the feedback of pain. One of the goals of all our interventions is to reduce stress. If an increase in cadence increases pain somewhere, you probably need to wonder if it is appropriate at this time. From her experience, Douek says to particularly pay attention to hamstring pain. "You could have some hamstring pain after a run—you're going to use your hamstrings in running," she says, so all pain isn't traceable to lifting too quickly. "But if the pain is high, right under the fold of the glute, that is problematic."

Two new devices can also help. The Stryd power meter measures how much energy you are using at any given moment. Wearing it, you can see your power output go down at the same pace when you run more efficiently. And you can see when it reverses and goes up at the same pace when you exceed an effective step rate for you. In my case, it shows me becoming more efficient, using less power at the same pace when I increase from high 160s to low 170s at a comfortable training pace. But when I approach or exceed 180—unless I'm running at about a 5K racing pace—my power score starts to climb back up. For now, I'm comfortable somewhere around 174. Note the "for now"—like all measures, this may—and will—change as my body and habits change.

Another tech tool, the Lumo Run, can also provide some guidance. A pod that clips on your waist and communicates with your phone, it measures cadence but also measures other important stride variables such as braking, bounce, pelvic rotation, and drop. As we've discussed, all of these work together to create an efficient stride. If you find that the other variables are strongly in the suggested "good" range, you probably can be assured that your cadence is okay, even if it hasn't reached the target goal.

The bottom line is that cadence is important, and increasing it can help with goals of injury prevention and performance enhancement. But it can't fix things all by itself. In fact, trying to increase cadence without first working on other elements can cause harm. The optimal cadence also varies by pace and for each individual—don't get caught up in trying to reach an "ideal" or comparing to others around you. Play with change, let your body adapt to new patterns, and in the end, listen to your body and learn to trust yourself.

9
MIX IT UP

VARIABILITY: THE ESSENTIAL CATALYST FOR IMPROVEMENT

IN THE LAST FEW CHAPTERS we've looked at systems that often get knocked out of whack due to our lifestyles and examined ways that we can both improve our mobility and correct imbalances. Often people will stop here, or proceed to cues that will hopefully help them incorporate new patterns and strengths. More important, however, and more effective than any cues, is using our body's innate abilities to choose and optimize our preferred movement paths.

Remember the stream flowing down the mountain, finding the path of least resistance between the contours of that particular slope? This is roughly the process that our bodies take in forming our preferred movement path, only it's more complex as the variables are greater, the body is smart, and it has memory.

The body has the remarkable capacity to recruit muscles in an endless variety of subtly changing patterns to achieve a similar end. So not only are the dimensions and properties of each individual's limbs, joints, and muscles unique, but the preferred methods of locomotion are unique as well. They are developed over time by a process called "plasticity."

Irish performance scientist John Kiely explains this process: "We first learn to move in ways shaped around our individually unique neurological and anatomical architectures. The more we move, the more we converge on favored solutions to individually specific problems."

In other words, we find what works for us, and over time, our brains and bodies ignore other options. Our movement patterns become deeply embedded, creating our unique, consistent running style. This conformity lets us become very efficient, using only the muscles required and letting others rest.

"Plasticity allows us to learn from the past experiences and to continually conform to previously successful movement solutions," Kiely says. "But then, it also encases us in a tomb of constraints—we get stuck in ruts."

REPETITIVE RUTS

Those ruts create two problems. One stems from the fact that variability serves as one of the key ways the body protects against injury. Even running on a track or treadmill, the body subtly varies each stride in complex patterns, spreading the work between different resources.

"The mechanical stress of running is distributed in ever-varying yet nonrandomly organized patterns," Kiely says. It's similar to how, each time you run on a trail, you step somewhere different while still following the direction of the trail and staying within boundaries, creating a wide, well-maintained path instead of a deep, narrow rut.

Studies, including a robust 2014 project by the Sports Medicine Research Laboratory in Luxembourg, have shown that lack of variability—running with exactly the same stride all the time—is highly correlated with injury. "Overuse injury is a lack of variability," says Kiely. "When variability goes down, you have the same tissues being hit the same way over time with no respite—that's the recipe for [an] overuse injury."

Variability goes down when the body becomes excessively fatigued. It also is reduced when we fail to vary the parameters of our runs. When we run the same way every day, we can do so mindlessly, shutting down not only the conscious mind but also the subconscious controller that adapts to changes. If we don't challenge the mind, it focuses its energies elsewhere, letting our running stride get increasingly static.

"Most of my injured patients either run on a treadmill all the time or run the same course over and over," says podiatrist Rob Conenello. "It's important to stress variability. Different shoes, different terrain, so you're not building up patterns. Change it around so you're not having problems. Run hills. Run on the trail."

Repetitive stress injuries aside, the neurological ruts we fall into due to lack of variability cause problems when we try to correct for imbalances or improve our stride efficiency. If we've been running with restricted hip flexors and sleeping glutes, our body's plasticity has found other ways to keep us upright and to propel us forward, and these ways have become normal for us. We've learned to move in inefficient, well-traveled ruts.

"We need to break out of those ruts," Kiely says. "And to do that we need to do something different."

Let's return to the analogy of the stream. The first time down the mountain, it flows into each valley and ravine, some of them dead ends, as it explores the easiest route down. Over time, however, the channel becomes deeper and narrower, eroded and entrenched into one option. Even when we create a new, more efficient route, the stream doesn't "look" for that route. It can't find it until the mountain gets shaken up—by an earthquake or a flood—and the exploration process starts again.

Similarly, when we change the parameters of our bodies' capacity, we need to shake up the system and loosen the ruts so new patterns can emerge. "You change resources," Kiely says. "But then you have to point those enhanced resources out to the central nervous system and convince the central nervous system that actually this is a better way to do it. Change proprioception, change strength, change tissue capacity—then it's got to be shaken up."

THE SPICE OF LIFE

Variability is the missing link in many runners' routines. More important than anything else discussed in this book, it's the first step to running better. Even without doing any corrective stretches or exercises, without cueing and form changes, variation will allow your body and brain to find better ways of moving.

"The most important thing for a runner is you have to mix up the signal, have to mix up their training," says podiatrist and biomechanist Simon Bartold. "Elites know about this. But your average runner in Manhattan will run in the same track in the same direction the same way every single time they run—and wonder why they get injured. You have to mix up the signal."

Even though variety is important at all times, it is especially essential when you're working to change and improve your running movements. After improving your range of motion and key strengths, you have to do something different to get your body to start using new patterns, or you'll simply keep running the same way. The magic is that when you shake things up and get the brain to pay attention again, it will find new patterns that are best for your mechanics. While there are some form cues that can help you consciously focus this process, substantial, effective change will occur subconsciously through the process of plasticity.

The most basic variation is pace. Simply running faster some days and slower on others is going to improve your stride. Different paces use different ranges of motion, different cadences, and different muscular stresses. Follow a training program that calls for a variety of different workouts: long runs, tempo runs, intervals at 5K pace, recovery runs, pure-speed workouts. If that is too ambitious for the mind-space you can devote to running right now, add strides to your routine 2 or 3 times per week (see page 134 for details on doing strides).

As discussed in the previous chapter, changing cadence can also alter stride mechanics and require sufficient focus to create new pathways and patterns. Make gradual changes so that the changes come naturally and gradually, not major modifications that might be unprofitable or injurious, such as trying to match an unrealistically high cadence.

You can, and should, also vary the terrain you run on. Even getting off the sidewalk and onto the grass or dirt beside it greatly enhances the variability of each foot plant and requires your body and mind to adapt to and explore new ways of moving. "Jump on an off-road path—just pop off the road," says professor of kinesiology Ryan Green, citing the benefits: "You have to be aware of the ground, your proprioception. You're doing core strength and drills and don't even know it."

Runners who are used to the road often balk at this, because it requires more focus and effort to run on trails than on a smooth, paved path. That is the point. The more challenging the terrain, the more the body and brain will focus, and that focus is required to start to rewire the system.

"It's doing something different physically, but also doing challenges that are sufficiently engaging that you have to actually zero in on them. You have to focus intently on them," Kiely says. "That's the catalyst for the slow change in brain chemistry that enables the plasticity channels in the brain."

The brain won't commit the resources to this process if it doesn't sense adequate challenge. "It has to be engaging," Kiely says. "The brain has to focus: 'This is the relevant stuff—if I don't get it right, there is a consequence.' Our brain will respond to what it feels is important."

When Kiely describes this, it sounds like what psychologist Mihalyi Csikszentmihalyi, PhD, calls "flow." Flow is the state where challenge equals skill, so that the task requires your full physical and mental focus—but doesn't exceed what you are able to accomplish. Often in running, the physical effort brings us to that focus. In this instance, we're looking for a coordination challenge at the precise level that we need in order to give it our full focus while not feeling overwhelmed so that we withdraw and make excuses.

To this end, fast-paced running down a technical trail may be one of the best ways to shake up your stride. Fast enough that you can't break your focus for 1 second, but not so fast that you're out of control.

Lacking access to steep, technical terrain several times a week, some, like Olympic sprint coach Dan Pfaff, introduce arbitrary and random variables to provoke rapid change and require intent focus. Pfaff has been known to draw irregularly spaced lines using chalk or tape on a sidewalk or track and to have runners go through them at a rapid pace. Andreas Behm, coach of Olympic hurdlers, uses horizontal ladders and low hurdles ("wickets") as obstacles to force athletes to disrupt ingrained running patterns. "Once athletes have stabilized a pattern, we oftentimes switch up spacings or even omit wickets at the end to continually introduce a new element to a familiar task," Behm says.

Andrew Kastor has the Mammoth Track Club runners do repeats in spikes in a grassy park that is not perfectly groomed, intentionally ensuring that they encounter holes, rough patches, uneven turns, and other obstacles that require reaction and adjustments in their strides.

"At a reasonable pace, the runner has to change cadence and stride length based on visual information, while maintaining speed," says Kiely. "If [you do it] too slowly, it's too easy: You don't have to focus. If [you] do it too quickly, you're bordering on risky."

More informally, I watch high school kids splash each other using the puddles along the roads during their easy days. It's a game to them, but it creates many of the elements desired: quick steps outside of the normal stride path for both the splasher and splashee, who has the added benefit of having to react without prior planning in which direction or speed. At other times they'll kick a rock along ahead of the group, each runner taking turns when it comes closest to him. They'll jump over benches, bushes, and playground equipment, push off the sides of rocks or walls. On special days, we'll hold an Ultimate Frisbee game, which has the team sprinting, turning, juking—barefoot on the football field. The key is to be creative, have fun, and challenge the kids to move in new ways.

During the months when I first focused on improving my posture and glute activation, my testing ground was a 400-meter segment about one-half mile from the end of most of my runs. This segment was slightly uphill over variable terrain on a twin-track jeep road. I would run it close to all out a couple times per week, focusing on staying tall and keeping everything connected.

The terrain was appropriately rough and variable underfoot. During dry spells, it would get sandy and deep. After a rain, the surface was firm but flaky, with washed-out gullies. Various weeds would encroach on the path. Not knowing if the next foot strike would be firm or soft, level or falling away, kept my strides quick and my ground contact short. I couldn't risk getting off balance and slipping on a patch of sand or falling into a hole. The speed was adequate to require all of my focus, and the distance was long enough to show me where I would fall apart if I wasn't focused on keeping everything tight and quick. I knew I was making progress when I could run the full 400 meters and feel like I was powering through it, not straining or flailing. Eventually I began to note these new mechanics spilling into all of my runs.

Research by Steve McGregor, PhD, and others at Eastern Michigan University suggests that simply pushing yourself harder, ideally keeping up with a fast group, is the one prerequisite for achieving a more economical style. "When you run against people who push you to run faster, you find the optimal way to run that speed—or you don't," McGregor explained to Matt Fitzgerald in a 2014 interview for *Competitor* magazine. "Running is so complex that it's difficult to put all of the pieces of the puzzle together consciously. The only thing you have to do consciously is try to run fast, and then the pieces of technique required to do that fall into place unconsciously."

Shoe Fetish

One final source of variety that many runners balk at is footwear. We tend to find a shoe model that fits and feels right, and we wear it every day until it wears out. But different shoes change how your foot interacts with the ground and allow your nervous system to play with your stride, allowing for adaptation. "The easiest way to change your movement pattern is to change your shoe," says podiatrist and advisor to the American Running Association Paul Langer.

Conenello says, "The best thing to tell people is to change your shoes every day." That sounds like a lot of shoes, but even a two-shoe rotation will help. You can have one lighter, more minimal shoe and one that's somewhat heavier and more cushioned. Or one with a slightly different heel-toe drop. Or a trail shoe and a road shoe—providing you get on the trails at least a couple times per week.

The biggest, and most effective, variation you can produce in footwear is to go without. Very few people advocate going barefoot all the time anymore, but there are a lot of things you can do while barefoot that will create variety in your stride, strengthen your feet, cue balance, and encourage a light, quick touchdown.

DRILLING FOR NEW PATTERNS

In addition to variety in your running routine, adding what people call "form drills" engages muscles, increases your range of motion, and creates movement patterns outside of your normal running stride. Doing these regularly while working on the flexibilities and strengths discussed in earlier chapters will help trigger the desired changes and integrate the new capabilities into your stride.

More effective than consciously cuing stride changes, drills work at the muscular and nervous system level to convince the body to try new movement paths. "There's not a lot of pedagogic step-by-step teaching," coach Bobby McGee says about improving form. "You address the range of motion, you address the strength deficits, you get drills to provide the balance and the rhythm and the skill, and then they organically move into the kind of running form that they were capable of when they didn't have environmental restrictions."

Here are several universally recommended integrative exercises and drills to help you mix things up, with suggestions on what to focus on and when to do them.

STRIDES

Strides are one of the simplest ways of improving your neuromuscular connections. They improve your running economy—teaching your body to move faster with less effort—as well as your maximum speed.

In his book, *Running Science*, Owen Anderson, PhD, explains that the pace you are able to sustain at any distance is a percentage of your maximal running speed. If you can improve your max speed over short distances, you will be able to sustain a faster pace when you run longer. Max speed is more about coordination than power.

"Maximal speed improves as the nervous system learns to coordinate the muscles in ways that promote faster stride rates, shorter contact times per step, and quicker generation of substantial propulsive forces," Anderson writes.

"Going all out is like turning a fire hose on full," says elite coach and author Brad Hudson. "It recruits every nerve and muscle group, including ones that don't often get used."

- **TO DO STRIDES:** After you've warmed up or at the end of your run, "Go as quick as you can—while staying relaxed," Hudson says. Focusing on maintaining a smile or a relaxed face can help keep you from straining. Stay tall, aim for a quick turnover, and push your stride out behind you, not reaching forward.

- Once you hit your top speed, shut it down as soon as you start to feel it takes any effort to maintain. Pushing too long—any longer than 10 to 12 seconds—will kick in your anaerobic energy system and increase acidity in your cells, which changes the workout. Plus, you'll start pacing yourself, or your stride will fall apart after a short burst, and the point is to shock the system with an all-out, coordinated effort. Your speed burst should happen so quickly that your heart rate and breathing don't have time to react.

- Slow to an easy walk and rest for a few minutes after each burst. Don't start another fast segment until your heart rate has dropped to close to a resting pulse—so you're ready for another maximum burst of nerves and muscle. Your last burst should feel as easy and be as fast as the first.

- If you're just starting, try 1 to 3 fast efforts per training session. As you feel more comfortable, add more, building up to 8 to 10 bursts. Some runners hit their top speed every day, but most of us only need to do strides 2 or 3 times per week.

- More advanced athletes do these sprints up a steep hill to maximize muscle recruitment and the shaking up of stride mechanics.

Barefoot Strides

Taking off your shoes to do strides on grass is a tried-and-true, highly effective way to cue new stride mechanics, which long outdates the last decades' minimalist and barefoot movements. Studies, like a 2014 investigation at Trinity College in Dublin, show that many people run differently shod and unshod. Full-time unshod running is practical only for a few, but if the goal is to shake up how you run, there are few better ways than to take off your shoes.

Mark Cucuzzella, who teaches healthy running courses around the country, recommends a progression, starting with soft, gentle, two-leg hops and gradually working up to all-out sprints.

- **TO DO BAREFOOT STRIDES:** Do 10 easy hops forward, then 10 back. Advance to a short one-leg hop. Then, with a very light, low stride, gently jog for 30 to 50 yards, noting how your foot lands and how your knees bend and hips move. Increase your turnover to hit an easy, long-run pace. Try a field length at 5K pace. If you're comfortable, run a few strides, going as fast as you can turn over without straining.

- Even after you've worked up to doing 8 to 10 strides all out, continue to do some barefoot work at other paces to encourage the neuromuscular recruitment in a barefoot running pattern at those paces. As noted above, sprinting is great for shaking things up and activating the full array of nerves and muscles, but most runners use a different stride when sprinting than they do when running long on the road— I've seen runners go from a tall, light barefoot sprint to a hunched, compromised distance stride without translating any of the movement pattern.

- When you return to your shoes and socks, put them on while standing up. This introduces single-leg balancing (the next drill) in a natural, contextual way.

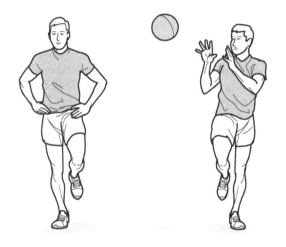

SINGLE-LEG BALANCE

Cucuzzella, biomechanists Jay Dicharry and Benno Nigg, and other experts all consider the ability to balance on one leg a prerequisite to running well. Kiely says, "Single-leg balance. That stuff is gold. Especially for high-mileage runners doing most at a similar pace." The exercise is as simple as it sounds.

- **TO DO THE EXERCISE:** After getting tall and balanced, with your weight equally on the balls of your foot and your heels, lift one foot off the ground and hold it in the air beneath you while you stand on the other. Stay balanced, without excessive wobbling, for 30 seconds. When you can do that, try it with your eyes closed. This removes the visual balancing cues and forces you to rely on the perceptions coming from your feet and muscles.

- With your eyes open, try tossing a ball back and forth with a partner. When you get better at balancing, make it a 6- to 8- pound medicine ball. Other ideas: While standing and balancing, put on your socks and shoes. Standing tall on one leg, drive the other foot back as if slamming a door behind you while keeping your torso straight—this both works balance and cues glute activation. "Any type of perturbation is activating the nervous system," Kiely says.

Dicharry says this type of nervous system training is better done in short 20- to 30-second segments several times a day rather than in one big block of time. So find times and events to prompt yourself to do it: when brushing your teeth, when you take your first sip of morning coffee, when you're waiting for a bus, when you take your first sip of afternoon coffee. You have to integrate it and do it regularly. The good news is that you can make rapid progress, with big changes in a few weeks, as neuro-muscular training is faster than building new muscles or stretching tight tendons.

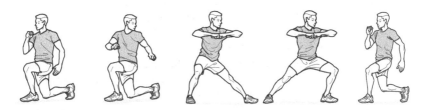

LUNGE MATRIX

The lunge matrix, recommended by a wide variety of coaches and therapists, combines numerous stretches and strength moves into one easy-to-remember circuit. You can do it before or after your run, but many recommend using it as the first thing you do for a warmup. "The goal of the lunge matrix is to reset your range of motion in all of the planes of movement," says Cucuzzella. In addition to affecting your range of movement, the matrix also activates muscles you've been working on like the glutes max and med and gets them ready to engage during your run.

Elite coach Jay Johnson says, "After 3 weeks of doing the lunge matrix before your runs, you'll not think of taking your first running step until you've gone through the routine; you simply feel better, more athletic when you run."

Initially developed by physical therapist Gary Gray, the 3D Dynamic Lunge Matrix includes five different lunges. Doing five sets for each leg brings you to 50 lunges for the full matrix—you can complete it in 3 to 5 minutes.

- **TO DO A FRONT LUNGE:** Take a strong step forward with your left foot, as far as you are tall, far enough that you can lower your right knee close to the ground while keeping your left thigh parallel to the ground and knee over your foot. Return to an upright position. Repeat with your right foot. Do 5 reps for each foot.

- **TO DO A FRONT LUNGE WITH A TWIST.** Repeat the front lunge, but when you are in the lowest lunge position, rotate your upper body 90 degrees toward the extended leg. If you are lunging with your left leg forward, your right shoulder will rotate toward your left knee. Do 5 reps for each foot.

- **TO DO A SIDE LUNGE:** With feet square, lift your right leg and step straight out to the right. Lower your body down as if sitting in a chair, with your right leg under your body and your left leg extended straight. Try to not let your right knee go any farther forward than your toes. Pressing back to an upright position, balance on both legs and then step to the left. Do 5 reps for each foot.

- **TO DO A 5 AND 7 O'CLOCK:** Take a big step back and to the side with your left leg, and place your foot down at 90 degrees from your left foot at the 5 o'clock position if you were standing on a clock face. Keeping your posture erect, lower your body over your left ankle. Your right leg will be straight, and you'll feel a stretch in the right hamstring. Push back to a neutral position and repeat with your right leg reaching back to the 7 o'clock position. Do 5 reps for each foot.

- **TO DO A BACKWARD LUNGE:** Lift your right leg and drive it straight backwards until your right knee is close to the ground and your left knee is over your left ankle with your left thigh parallel to the ground. As you lift your right foot to return, drive it upward with your glute, then pull it forward and through so that your right heel skims your butt. Repeat with your left leg driving back. Do 5 reps for each foot.

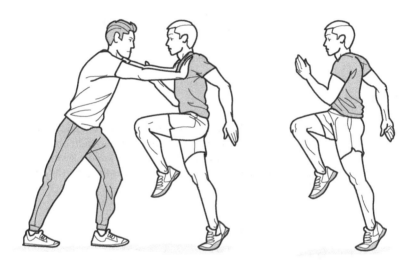

HIGH KNEES

One of the most common form drills, high knees exaggerates the stride and activates the glute on the supporting leg. It develops a full range of motion and quick ground contact time.

Coach McGee points out that many runners lean back when they do high knees, looking like a drum major. He considers this a fatal flaw, reinforcing the action of contracting the hip flexor (front of the hip) rather than stretching and loading it with hip extension and the knee coming forward as an elastic unloading reaction. To correct this, he recommends pairing up with a partner, ideally of similar height.

- **TO DO THE DRILL:** Your partner will stand facing you with his or her hands on both of your shoulders. Leaning slightly into your partner's hands, push forward, driving each leg down firmly into the ground and letting the other rebound up to close to a 90-degree angle with the body, but no higher. Don't force the knee up—focus on driving with the support leg and quick, light steps. Once your posture is set, the partner can step away and you can continue the drill, moving forward for 20 to 50 meters.

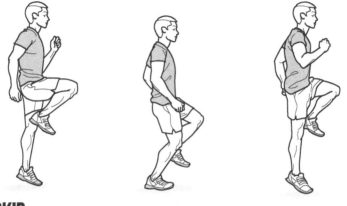

A-SKIP

The popular A-Skip is similar to high knees, adding a quick skipping motion on the support leg with each stride. This adds to the coordination challenge and encourages quick ground contact time. As with high knees, keep your posture tall and focus on the downward drive of the leg rather than trying to lift your knees as high as possible.

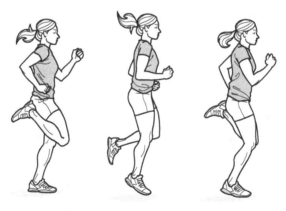

BUTT KICK

This drill exaggerates the backward drive and heel lift during the swing phase of your stride, engaging the glutes and hamstrings and stretching the quads.

- **TO DO THE DRILL:** Stand tall with your hips square and your weight on the balls of your feet. Drive one leg back so that the heel comes up toward your buttocks. As that foot is coming back beneath you, kick the other leg up toward your butt. Try to relax your muscles so that you actually touch your heel to your butt, but don't strain. Move forward gradually in a quick, quiet shuffle for 20 to 50 meters.

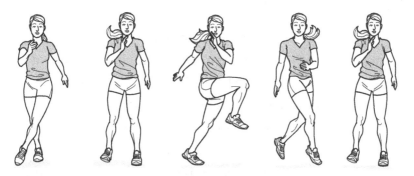

CARIOCA

This sideways-stepping move works the muscles on the inside and outside of your hips and helps with balance and reducing ground contact time.

- **TO DO THE DRILL:** Start by bringing your right leg behind your left leg, then drive your left leg out farther to the left. Bringing your right knee up, drive it in front and across your left leg, then drive your left leg again out to the left. Continue alternating front and back for 20 to 50 meters.

- Facing the same direction, return, now moving your left leg behind and in front of your right leg.

- Try holding your arms out straight while you do this. This cues the core activation necessary to keep your torso straight while your legs move and create torsional forces. It also helps keep your attention on the drill and the muscles being used.

BACKWARD RUNNING

Striding backward is a great way to activate your glutes, as it is difficult to perform without using them.

- **TO DO THE DRILL:** Start by simply lifting one leg and reaching it backward, then the other, walking a few steps. Feel the glute working to lift rather than the hip flexor in front. Advance to a run, reaching your leg out as far as you can behind you without bending forward or arching your back. Go 20 to 50 meters. Turn around and return, running backward, taking short steps as quickly as you can turn your feet over.

Lunge-Balance Sequence

If the list of drills and exercises gets overwhelming, you need not give up and do nothing. I've been there and felt like I needed to take a list out to remind me what to do next—which I never did—so I ended up doing whatever I remembered, rather haphazardly. Another way is to create a sequence that flows naturally from pose to pose, making it easy to remember and quick to perform.

Working with physical therapist Trent Nessler, natural-running expert Cucuzzella, and kinesiologist and coach Green, we devised a sequence. "This is especially effective for those under time constraints for their workout," Green says. It takes approximately 5 minutes to complete 10 sets. (We timed it.)

This sequence reinforces several key elements of an efficient stride, specifically hip and glute strength, hip and shoulder flexibility, and dynamic balance.

Move through the exercises smoothly and slowly before and/or after every run, or at other times during the day. Hold each position for 1 to 2 seconds.

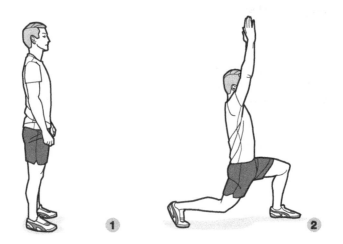

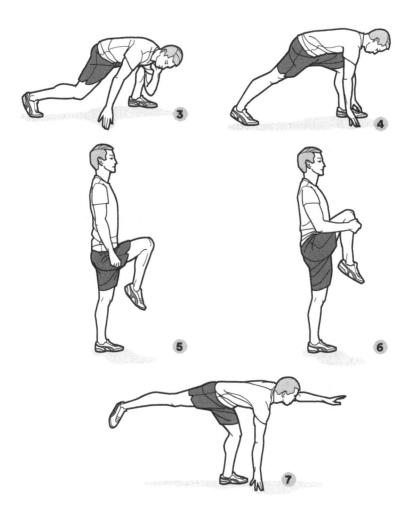

1. Start by standing tall, with your weight balanced on the balls and heels of both feet.

2. Step into a lunge with your left foot forward and with your knee tracking straight over your second toe and not extending forward past your foot. Raise both arms as if reaching for a high shelf above your head, rotating your pelvis back and stretching your right hip flexor as you focus your upper body on being straight and tall.

3. Sink down and place your right hand on the ground to the right of your front foot. Bring your left arm over your left knee and lower it to touch the inside of your left ankle with your left elbow. In this position, straighten your right knee, contract your right glute, and drive your right hip forward.

4. Bring your left hand back over your knee and place both hands on the ground in track starting position. Rock your weight to your back leg, getting the heel down toward the ground and stretching your right calf and left hamstring.

5. As you straighten to a standing position, first drive your right leg back, then swing your right leg forward and up. Pause briefly in balanced running pose with your right thigh parallel to the ground.

6. Grab your right knee with your right hand and your shin with your left hand and pull upward toward your right shoulder to stretch your glute.

7. Rotate your right leg down and back, then straighten and lift it behind you while you drop your upper body to a horizontal position and reach down with your right hand to touch the ground to the right of your left foot.

8. Step into a lunge with your right foot forward, swinging your arms over your head.

Repeat the sequence 8 to 10 times on each side.

10
THE JOURNEY

BUYING INTO THE NEED FOR CHANGE
AND CREATING NEW LIFESTYLE HABITS

IF YOU'VE MADE IT THIS far into this book, you obviously care about your running and want to do it better. Whether or not you'll actually implement any of the advice, do the work, and make changes is still very iffy, though. Most people do not.

Being world-class at denial and avoidance myself, I'm too often happy to continue my current patterns with just a nagging sense that I should be making changes and might be heading off a cliff. I can speak expertly to the many reasons why people don't change.

I believe the cardinal reason for resisting the work of improving our form stems from the fact that most of us don't have to change to keep running. The body is stunningly resilient at finding ways to keep functioning despite all the crap we put it through. "Because of the remarkable capacity of the human body to compensate, we get away with things for quite a while," says podiatrist Ray McClanahan.

And that may be okay. We all have lives outside of running, and running serves many different functions in different people's lives. "It's a bit of a journey," former elite runner Grant Robison says. "No matter how many studies you read or whatever somebody says to you, if you're not in a place where you really want to change your form, I don't think it would be good to change it."

As a coach, I've found that nothing I say makes a bit of difference until a runner decides to focus on this part of his running. "You have to arrive at that place on your own," says Robison. "If you're not ready to embrace the focus to get dialed in, it just becomes a headache, a bother."

Before you set sail on that journey, here are some reasons you may resist boarding the boat, and some thoughts on how to make it across the gangway and enjoy a successful trip.

HIJACKING THE ESCAPE POD

One of the primary reasons adult, nonprofessional runners get out the door is for the mental release of running. Running is our escape, our time to *not* focus, monitor, and analyze, but instead let our minds drift and relax.

I described one aspect of this in a recent *Runner's World* column.

> *As duties and deadlines mount while phones buzz, emails ping, news and Twitter feeds and colleagues and family and friends all demand attention, I feel a growing panic that I can't keep up. The world is sweeping past and time is slipping away—there's not enough of it to accomplish what I have to do, let alone do what I want.*
>
> *And then I pull on shorts and running shoes and head out on the road. Within a mile, with distractions removed and panic hormones flushed from my veins, I slow to a sustainable rhythm. I settle into the present activity, not mentally rushing into the future. I see, as Annie Dillard wrote*

in Pilgrim at Tinker Creek, *"that this is it, and find it world enough, and time." Suddenly things that were urgent no longer seem important. Problems that were unsolvable fall into place. Large projects become manageable. I realize that I lack not hours but focus. Time stretches out as endless as a childhood summer. I have only to choose how to use it.*

I am the first to admit that this feeling, this escape, can be a far cry from the thoughts and feelings of a run where I am focused on my form.

That run might go like this.

Within a mile, I note that my shoulders are still hunched forward, as if over my laptop. I pull them back, fighting the tightness in my chest. My back and sides feel strained from my unpracticed upright posture. My Garmin beeps the mile split, and as I check it, I see that my cadence is in the low 160s. I try to speed it up and note that I'm reaching too far forward. This sends my attention to my hips, which are clearly tight and tilted. I get tall, feel my hips rotate and my glutes kick in, and for a few minutes I'm running quietly and smoothly, but somewhat slower. I relax and drift mentally, finding some peace and escape in the run—until I pass a storefront and see my reflection. It shows I'm back in the compromised, sitting position I've had since 1977, and I quickly return my focus to my form.

The comparison is stark, and it's easy to see why we need to be overwhelmingly convinced the latter scenario is worthwhile before we give up a minute of the freedom a run can provide. We run for many reasons, and the time to escape and meditate is precious. You don't want to spend all of that time obsessing over matters like posture and stride frequency.

While that concern is legitimate, and you do need to be prepared to spend some of your runs somewhat constrained by a new mental focus, it need not take over every run forever. You will eventually learn the new patterns, and while you'll need to continue to be careful that your life outside of running doesn't sabotage your new mobility and strengths, you will find the stride changes can become default and permanent.

"If you restore the body to balance, then everything works fine," sports rehab specialist and coach Laura Bergmann says. "You don't have to think about hip extension, you don't have to think about where [you're] going to put [your] foot—because the body is now stacked naturally and all that can happen."

Besides the fact that the alternative would be worse—being injured and not being able to run at all—the distraction of form training also needs not be as bad as I've described. While Chapter 12 presents a few form cues that you can apply on your run, particularly as you fatigue, the majority of the process has to occur unconsciously, letting your body optimize as you give it new possibilities. You can't, in fact, think about these things too much or you'll likely force something unnatural.

Runners have long known this. "Don't worry too much about having to remember all these points about running form," Bob Glover wrote nearly 20 years ago in *The Competitive Runner's Handbook*. "Learning good running form is largely second nature."

Coach Bobby McGee says when people come along who are very right-brained and want to force the process, it reminds him of the story of the Nepalese guru trying to teach enlightenment to Westerners. "The guru says, 'It will take 5 years.' 'What if I work really hard?' asks the eager apprentice. 'Then it will take 10 years,' says the guru."

The methods for helping the mind and body rewire themselves—such as running fast over variable terrain, going barefoot, doing drills—may be different than your typical, mindless running fix, but they can also be fun and distracting. And you don't need to do them every day: In the course of mixing things up, many of your workouts can and should just be runs.

Given the body's ability to optimize its patterns, the process of change can be less invasive than we may have been led to believe. The discipline to do the necessary stretches and strength work is another matter. Most runners love to run—so much so that I've often told people who are impressed with my "discipline" that running for me is play, even a vice. We are unaccustomed to forcing ourselves to do mundane exercises that are good for us. And many of us have not been convinced that we need to.

A RUNNER, NOT AN ATHLETE

In 1993, Philadelphia Phillies first baseman John Kruk, when chided for behavior unbecoming an athlete, famously quipped, "I ain't an athlete, lady, I'm a ballplayer."

Kruk's unathletic status was reinforced by his "Ruthian" physique, which didn't prevent him from becoming a three-time All-Star and leading the Phillies to the World Series that year, thanks to his proficiency at one skill: swinging the bat.

Despite having a decidedly different physique than Kruk, I've always related to his quote. More than once, I've said some version of, "I'm not an athlete, I'm a runner." I've never had an athlete's strength, speed, or agility—just a slight build, a tenacious spirit, and a willingness to suffer. Those assets were enough to get me a spot on the varsity cross-country team throughout high school and to make me a serious local/regional competitor for most of my life.

I, like most, assumed that the best runners were just born that way. Like Kruk, I also felt that anything I might do to make myself more "athletic" was not only irrelevant but likely counterproductive. I don't need muscles that will weigh me down, just lungs and heart, physically and emotionally.

International runner and author Roger Robinson, PhD, now competing as a veteran in his late seventies, said something similar a few months ago. Telling me about rehabbing his new artificial knee, he said he told the nurse at one point, "I know what you're doing—you're trying to give me a core! I've never had a core in 50 years of running!" Roger is old school, from an era when you ran hard and long and not only didn't build a core but you didn't lift weights or stretch much either. Even so, he is now having to build a core, much to his chagrin.

"Runners in general are notoriously not very strong people," says podiatrist Rob Conenello. "When [we] start out, we are the skinny kids. We didn't like doing bench press, because we could only bench 90 pounds." We're the ones who didn't make the cut on the other sports teams. This carries over. We don't like strength or do strength.

As a doctor, however, Conenello's seen that getting stronger, no matter where you start, is essential for both injury prevention and performance. "Best thing I've learned: Everyone has to be stronger," he says. "A stronger runner is a better runner. We're not strong enough. It means making your foot stronger, your core stronger, instead of just going out there and running."

The Engine versus the Drive Train

But going out there and running is easier, and it feels far more productive. No amount of drills, weights, or yoga will replace the simple act of wearing off the bottom of your running shoes. Running fast is a function of the size of your engine—how much power you can generate over time—and the efficiency of your drive train. Improving your engine will allow you to run better than most, even if you're rolling on a less-than-ideal drive train.

"You can be a good runner and not be good at running," Robison says. "Vice versa, you can be a very slow runner and be very good at running—in terms of being very efficient." Seeing this, it's no wonder people gravitate toward simply running more.

In my coaching, I've also noted that there seems to be a dichotomy in runners' thinking between their ability to alter their performance and their form. Performance is seen as something you can work toward through training and repetition, while form feels innate and difficult, if not impossible to change. Any work on it feels stilted, arbitrary, and uncomfortable.

I've found runners are more likely to do squats than shoulder mobility work. They'd rather be running, but doing squats at least makes them feel like they are building strength for running. Plus, they *are* work: You feel strain in your muscles, you sweat, your heart rate goes up. It beggars belief that balancing on one foot, doing toe yoga, or even holding a static hip flexor stretch can make much of a difference in your running ability.

Besides feeling too far removed from the effort of running, the formwork, while it doesn't strain your systems, is surprisingly difficult. "As simple as we can make it, in the end it is not that easy," Robison says about formwork. "People try it and realize it does take a lot of work."

"You need to invest," says Rebecca Shultz of Lumo Bodytech. "If biomechanical improvement is your goal, it is going to take some time. You're going to have to do work." While runners tend to accept that getting faster requires an investment in both effort and time, form seems to be considered something that can be fixed instantly.

"People want success overnight—we live in a society where everyone's looking for a silver bullet, the quick fix," Shultz says. "When it comes to something like improving running form or losing weight—any physical change in your body—it takes time."

Worse Before Better

Not only does it take disciplined focus and time, but modifying your form will make all of your running harder at first. "Anything that deviates from a runner's preferred pattern increases metabolic energy costs," podiatrist Paul Langer says. "You'll feel like you're running slower and working harder." It requires a lot of faith to accept a setback and trust that this will eventually make you a better runner.

"It feels very uncomfortable before it feels comfortable," says Shultz. "You're changing your muscular recruitment patterns, you're building strength, you're trying to create new muscle memory. Your brain has to readjust and rewire. These things all take a little bit of time. They're not something you can do in a week and expect it to work for you. Certainly it is going to hurt. [It is going] to be uncomfortable. It's hard to convince someone that it is going to be awful, but it will get better."

But to anyone paying attention, it is increasingly clear that just doing miles and becoming a stiff, single-strength runner won't make you the best. The best in the world at every level spend considerable effort on mobility and strength to give them an edge beyond their gifted abilities. It isn't a matter of either building the engine or improving the drive train, but both.

While you may decide not to focus in this area when you're a young, open-class athlete content with the performances you achieve with your current mechanics, every runner needs to take it more seriously as she ages. I've rarely met a masters runner who didn't consider mobility and strength work essential for surviving and succeeding in the upper age groups. "We compensate pretty well over a period of time, then get to the point where we can't," says McClanahan.

As I entered my mid-forties, I, like many others, quickly found that 25-plus years of running was taking its toll on my body in ways I had never anticipated. A more serious approach to core strength, form, and range-of-motion drills has cured all of the new aches and has made me feel stronger and fitter than ever. It also makes me wonder what more I might have been able to accomplish had I seen the light sooner in life. Do you have the foresight and discipline to find out before you start breaking down?

Even those who are converted to the idea of building athleticism as a runner, however, often still don't do much along this score. I can't, of course, look into the minds of each runner, but I've experienced and seen a few other things that contribute to our difficulty committing ourselves to this kind of work.

Can't Get No Satisfaction

The first hurdle runners have to overcome is the lack of feedback they get from supplementary work. Every run gives you the affirmation of distance and pace. You can easily chart your progress in workout and race times or keep track of your longest runs. But it is difficult to assess when you've gained another degree of flexibility in your hip. There are no Strava apps to report how long you spent doing squats and donkey kicks, and no one will be impressed with your toe splay ability.

"Working on your hip flexibility is not fun," says Robison. "There's nothing exciting or enjoyable about it." But getting up early on Saturday for a long run or doing a speed workout on the track like a 12 × 400m isn't fun or exciting to most people either, for that matter. The difference is that the run gives us an opportunity for the sense of flow. Flow, as explained by psychologist Mihalyi Csikszentmihalyi, occurs when we bring advanced skills to accomplish a difficult challenge. We get a sense of satisfaction when we can say, "This is really hard—but I can do it!" Every time we lace up and head out, we get a sense of competence, progress, even superiority. In contrast, while the supplementary work requires focus and time, it is hard to know if you're even doing a stretch or a drill correctly, let alone gaining skill.

No one I've talked to has a great solution for this problem. Coaches Andrew Kastor and Bergmann say people will see the improvement in their workout and race times. That is certainly great motivation. But then you wonder if the improvement was a result of the stretching or the extra intervals—it is probably both, but one feels more directly connected.

Others suggest taking photos or videos of your running to provide feedback on progress. While this can be useful, it is also risky. Runners may try to change their form in unnatural ways to conform to an ideal image. Like hearing the sound of our own voice, we rarely get to see our own running style. And mostly we'd like to avoid both: Just as we hate hearing our voice on a recording, we hate seeing video of us running. The reality differs from our perception and is often painful.

That doesn't mean we shouldn't look and learn both to accept reality as well as to use it as motivation to improve. But take note as well that, after doing flexibility and strength work, performance scientist John Kiely says, "You will be a more robust athlete, more resilient. But whether the change is visibly manifest is uncertain." Form changes tend to be subtle and take time to become evident.

Biomechanist Jay Dicharry and mobility expert Brad Cox advise doing regular assessments to provide feedback and show progress. It can be motivating to work toward the ability to execute a clean single-leg squat, for example. But it's hardly something you'd post to Facebook, like a half marathon PR, or brag about to training partners, like completing a killer workout.

In the end, Dicharry says, "I've become blunt enough that I'll sometimes say, 'Do you want to improve? Okay. Great. Here's what it takes.' If they don't want to follow the extra work, they are selling their performance potential short. That's their eventual decision—people need to supply their own motivation to get on board and take a trip."

A NEW NORMAL

Beyond the promise of improved performance or fewer injuries, I have found that runners who make the trip and get to a better place do find an intrinsic motivation to continue in how their body now feels.

Doing stretches and drills can become like brushing your teeth. Few adults achieve flow while brushing their teeth, or look for feedback that they are doing it well and getting better at it every day. No one posts tooth-brushing PRs. You also don't have to brush your teeth to accomplish your daily tasks—unlike getting dressed or eating breakfast, skipping tooth brushing won't get you arrested or make you weak and tired. But after you've become accustomed to the feeling of clean teeth, going without feels wrong: gross and unnatural.

Similarly, once you've opened up your hips and shoulders and learned to stand and stride more effectively, the new posture and balance feel good. Once you've strengthened and engaged your feet, you like their new dynamic, springy power. And it feels wrong, even gross like slimy teeth, when you stop the maintenance work and let daily sitting start to encroach on your posture again, or when your feet start to feel tired and sore, in need of heavy, supportive shoes. You find a new normal, one that allows you to move better, and you want to keep it.

NOT BROKEN, JUST HUMAN

To get to a point where supplementary work around our running becomes a part of our daily routine requires a shift in many people's approach to health and injury. Too often we hold a binary view: Either we're healthy and strong, or we're weak and broken. When we're healthy, we think we can handle anything, and not only do we have no need for maintenance but we also consider doing it a sign of weakness. A case in point is the high school runner who responds, "I'm not going to break," when I chide him about not doing his stretching. He misses the point.

This thinking leads to a pattern that surprises Robison, who sees it even among strong, fast runners. "People who are really good runners time-wise: It's incredible how they will get hurt, and they won't have any intention of changing anything other than just resting the injury, fixing it, then basically revving up, and repeating what they just did physically," Robison says. "They never stop and say, 'Let's work on different things.'"

Doing the same thing over and over and expecting a different result is commonly considered one of the definitions of insanity. To change, maybe we start to accept that injury is part and parcel of life, that the training process itself involves injury and recovery as we break down our bodies and let them rebuild themselves stronger. "We are wounded simply by participating in life, by being children of Adam and Eve," writes philosopher Thomas Moore in *Care of the Soul*. "To think that the proper or natural state is to be without wounds is an illusion."

If we start to accept that we're in a constant flux of health, that having gimpy hamstrings and tight lats are normal consequences of being alive and living in the 21st century, then maybe we can start working on them without feeling inadequate.

It can be as simple as changing your vocabulary. Kastor says he finds athletes have more trouble doing work that is described as "correctional"—as if they are broken and need to be repaired—as opposed to "ancillary"—something extra they are doing to add to their success. "'Correctional' puts you behind the eight ball. I'm wrong to begin with," Kastor says. "Ancillary training will boost your running."

I believe it would also help if we would rename "injury prevention" as "injury proofing." *Prevention* by its very name is a goal defined by the absence of something. *Proofing* can be seen as the process of making ourselves stronger so we become the invincible athletes we imagine ourselves to be. By changing our perception, maybe then we could see training elements like mobility, strength, and formwork as positive, forward-looking processes we put up front in our training.

"You want to improve your performance, you're putting all this work in," Bergmann says. "Why won't you spend 5 minutes to take a minute off your time? If you get in proper alignment, you will be faster. If I'm putting in all these miles, I'm going to do everything I can to ensure I'm getting the most out of those miles."

Runners want to set positive, motivational targets: Run more, run faster, set PRs, conquer new challenges. Advice on avoiding injury usually starts with not doing too much. But this is, again, a negative proposition. Sure, we can reduce injury by not pushing it, but we want to push it. The whole idea of training and racing is to blow past boundaries.

I think progress toward integrating ancillary work begins with seeing it not as avoiding something bad, but as an integral part of our training. Let's focus on what we can do to make ourselves ready for the challenges posed by our goals rather than scaling our aspirations—and our running—to our limited capabilities. Timing is everything. Yes, we get injured by doing too much, but just as often, it is because we first did too little.

FINDING TIME

"I get it," you say. But then you plead, "How can I do more? I simply don't have enough time." Without getting into a discussion about how much time we do or do not have, I understand the struggle. Adding something else that you have to schedule and plan and justify does often feel like too much.

There is no doubt that making these kind of changes requires time management. "To train smart movements, you need to do 4,000 to 6,000 reps to change your body's perception of what feels normal," Dicharry says. I did the math: If you do 20 reps in each session, that's 200 to 300 sessions, or once every day for 6 to 10 months. When it comes to new strengths, like in your glute med or foot arch, Dicharry says it requires working on it 2 to 4 days per week to improve, and then, once a desired level is achieved, 1 or 2 times per week to maintain.

McGee says that while duration creates strength—you can work longer during strength sessions to see benefits—it takes frequency to make skill. To improve neuromuscular patterns, you must work at it often. Frequency is important not only to learn the skill but to integrate it. Dicharry has seen many runners learn to use their hips in exercises but then instantly revert to old patterns as soon as they start running or whenever they speed up.

You have to make it part of who you are and how you move as a runner. In my years of coaching as well as running myself and observing runners, I've seen only two strategies that work to ensure the frequency and consistency necessary to make a difference.

Give Me 5 Minutes

The first strategy is to make a few elements mandatory, habitual, and an unconscious part of your running routine.

"Start with simple exercises to get the muscles *smarter* and do lots of reps. Every single day," Dicharry says in *Anatomy for Runners*. After a while, you'll start to feel a change: more mobility, an opening of the hips, the ability to contract new muscles, and the strength to hold new postures.

"Build the memory first, and then add another and another," Dicharry says. At some point, a lightbulb goes off. "Then you can work on cuing posture when you walk, stand, and even run," Dicharry says. "Just start simple."

A few years ago, after a bout of high hamstring pain, I started doing the lunge matrix before every run. Not just on hard workout days, not just days when I had more time, not just the days when I thought about it—every single day. I simply didn't run without first doing some lunges in all planes of motion. And I still don't. The same is now true of all the scholastic runners I coach.

Even on early morning workouts, they start by doing lunges whether or not a coach is there or anyone has prompted them.

This summer, I added three simple glute routines after the run and before stretching: squats, bridges, and side-leg lifts. We did the same ones and we did them every day. This violates the variety rule and the hard/easy rule, but adding them was changing our routine and the simplicity was essential for making it the new habit.

Since it was the off-season and none of our workouts was that intense, adding a few strength elements didn't overtax anybody, even on long days. I've found that trying to remember to do something 2 or 3 times per week usually means doing it once a week at best—when you remember that you've forgotten. By doing them every day, the runners soon incorporated them on their own, whenever they finished a run, not waiting for the coach to remind them.

Our pre- and postrun routines take 5 minutes at most. A few years ago, *Running Times* published a nice collection of mobility drills by Jay Johnson called "Give Me 15 Minutes." The exercises are all great—many similar to what is recommended in earlier chapters here—and 15 minutes, or more, is probably ideal. But I've found that even that much time and complexity is too much for many noncoached runners today.

"If folks have time, sure—those are great," says coach Ryan Green about such drill routines. "But if you think about the everyday runner, like a doctor we have here: He runs Boston in like 2:50, but he's an ER doc. His hours are crazy, he has very little time. Is he going to spend an extra 30 minutes doing these drills when his time is so limited? I would love to say yes, but chances are it is going to be no."

Better, then, to choose one or two and do them religiously than try to add a bunch and do them sporadically. Once the few have become habitual, you can switch them out or perhaps add a new one.

Another strategy that I've used and seen others incorporate is to create workouts that integrate various elements into a seamless process. For example, after lunges, the cross-country team will run a mile to the golf course (you could use a football field or a grassy park lawn as well). At the course, they take off their shoes and do toe spreads, short-foot exercises, and pull up grass with their toes. Then, still barefoot, they do a few form drills and run a turnover workout of short sprints up to 200 meters. Upon returning to their shoes, they put shoes and socks on while standing, using the difficulty of brushing grass off their feet as an added balancing challenge. We then run a longer course back to school. Making the barefoot strength and balancing elements part of the workout saves time and makes them more real and much easier to remember and accomplish than a list of separate, arbitrary tasks.

The lunge-balance sequence discussed in Chapter 9, which originated with Green, is another example of combining multiple exercises into one seamless, easy-to-remember sequence that you can do quickly and habitually.

Multitask

More important and more successful than adding elements to your running routine is the process of integrating posture, mobility, and strength work into your everyday life. You can work on many of these skills all day, every day.

Many people resist doing this, wanting instead to compartmentalize their running from the rest of their day. When I suggested that my high school–age son move his gaming screen higher up on his desk so he didn't have to slouch over it, he made it clear: "You can coach my posture while I'm running, but not when I'm playing video games." When I point out that students' shoulders are rotated forward because of being hunched over computers and cell phones, they say, "But that is the way we are, that is the way we are comfortable."

As a reader of this book, I assume you are beyond that (and you don't have the burden of being coached by your father). But even if you've bought in, it takes another level of commitment to decide that you are going to change how you move every hour you are awake—maybe even when you are sleeping. But not only does this allow you to find time in surprising and hidden spots, but it also is truly the only way to make some changes.

"If not life-integrated, doing [postural and mobility work] sporadically does not make the gains you want," says mobility expert Cox. "People say, 'I do it twice a week'—but what did you do for 50 hours at work?" There's just no way to spend most of the time reinforcing one pattern and correcting for it with 5 minutes here and there, and then think you can integrate that into your stride when you are running.

"If you're in a certain posture for 8 hours, there is no way you're going to run with a tall spine," says Bergmann. "People have to break it down, [saying, for example] 'I want to work on this thing: standing up straighter.' Even if you have restrictions, focusing on it will slow down the decline. Even whatever is straight for them. Just sit up straight and stand up straight all day. That will make a huge difference."

Most of the stretches and exercises described earlier can be integrated into your everyday life outside of running. Here are a few suggestions.

> **BALANCE ON ONE FOOT WHEN BRUSHING YOUR TEETH.** One of the most common suggestions seems almost too easy. This time is already scheduled and you likely don't need the mind space to focus on the act of brushing. The trick is remembering to do it early in the morning, and making it habitual.

> **BALANCE ON ONE FOOT WHILE PUTTING ON YOUR SOCKS AND SHOES.** Don't sit. Stand and balance on one leg while you reach for and pull on your sock, then your shoe. Stay balanced while you tie the laces. Then switch feet and repeat. Alternate which foot you start with, so that each day you're balancing barefoot on a different side.

> **DO GLUTE EXERCISES AS PART OF YOUR MORNING COFFEE OR TEA ROUTINE.** When I bought a hand-crank coffee grinder a few years ago, I started doing air squats during the time it took me to grind the beans. Now I can finish 15 to 20 squats while cranking enough for an espresso. It was the first time I was ever that consistent, and it made a huge difference in my glute strength and activation. Now I can't grind without doing squats. It's part of the same action in my mind.

> Caspar Coppetti, one of the founders of On shoes in Switzerland, does clamshells while his espresso is brewing. "I'd like to just drink the coffee," he says. But he tells himself, "If you don't do the clams, you don't get the coffee." He credits the resulting strength and form improvement with saving his running.

Be creative, but find something you'll do that doesn't require a decision everyday. Make it part of your quotidian routine.

❱ **SIT TALL WHILE DRIVING.** Even though you are sitting in the driver's seat, you can work on posture by sitting as tall as you can: Bring your chest and shoulders up, tighten your abs, and reduce the curve of your spine. Pull your head back and high. Set your rearview mirror for this height—every time you slouch, it will remind you by being out of line.

❱ **PULL YOUR SHOULDERS BACK AND RAISE YOUR HEAD HIGH EVERY TIME YOU SEE A CERTAIN COLOR OR WALK THROUGH A DOORWAY.** Athletes as excellent as world-champion marathoner Mark Plaatjes and Olympic medalist Deena Kastor use such mnemonic devices.

❱ **DO AB CONTRACTIONS OR SHORT-FOOT EXERCISES WHILE DRIVING.** When you get bored on a long drive, try contracting your TA muscle (the inner abdominal one between your hip bones) and holding it tight as long as you can, timing it with the dashboard clock. Or, with the cruise control on, do short-foot contractions.

❱ **PLAY WITH YOUR BALANCE AND HIP PROPRIOCEPTION WHILE STANDING IN LINE AT THE COFFEE SHOP.** Or when you are waiting for the subway, standing in line to board a plane, or waiting to order a sandwich. Essentially, any time you are standing, think about rotating your hips so they aren't spilling out the front and getting your balance over your feet, not locked back on the heel. Do it during the national anthem at your kid's Little League or basketball game. While you're at it, stay standing during the game if you can find an unobtrusive place, keeping good posture for as long as you can.

▶ CUE YOUR GLUTE ACTIVATION WHEN WALKING THE DOG. Any time you're walking you can consciously activate your glutes. Get tall and clench your butt on each side with each stride, pushing each leg back with a slightly exaggerated motion and landing beneath you, not reaching out in front.

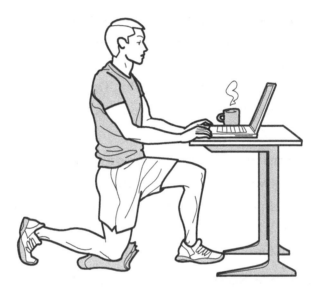

▶ DO HIP EXTENSION STRETCHES WHILE WORKING ON YOUR COMPUTER. Just push the chair to the side and kneel on one knee in front of your desk. Get your hip rotated and hold it while you check email. Five minutes per side goes quickly during the workday. You can do it 2 or 3 times: in the morning, after lunch, and during your final few, last-check minutes of the day.

▶ DO FOOT-STRENGTHENING EXERCISES AT YOUR DESK. Even with your shoes on, you can do the short-foot exercise or isometric pushes against the floor and the sides of the desk. Conenello suggests stretching the top of your foot and shin at your desk. They get tight from driving and always being held in a flexed position—bent toward the leg—rather than extended down and back. "Take your foot, put it behind you with [your] toes extended, and push down," he says. Or, he suggests, "Focus on pushing your big toe into the ground during a lecture." Add toe yoga and pick-up exercises any time you can take off your shoes under your desk.

❱ **DO A STANDING HIP STRETCH WHILE ON A CONFERENCE CALL.** Lift one leg onto your chair, make yourself tall, and push forward on the supporting hip. No one can see you, and it doesn't require heavy breathing. Or balance on alternating legs—just make sure you don't lose your balance, fall, and make a crash.

❱ **DO STRETCHES, BRIDGES, OR FOOT STRENGTHENING WHILE WATCHING TV OR READING IN THE EVENING.** It's private, it's downtime physically—you can do just about anything you want. You just have to get your butt off the couch. Use the couch for the couch hip flexor stretch (page 47) instead.

❱ **SQUAT WHENEVER YOU'D USUALLY BEND.** Rather than bending down from the waist, stick your butt out and lower into a squat when you're weeding the garden, picking strawberries, petting your dog, picking up the kids' toys, or rearranging the bottom bookshelf. Squatting feels like more work at first, but for extended tasks you quickly note how it moves the stress from your back to your glutes, and you're changing the way you move. Be careful to maintain good form, with your knees never extending in front of your toes. Your knees should not hurt and you should not force a squat.

❱ **WORK ON HIP EXTENSION WHILE SLEEPING.** If you sleep on your side, you likely pull both legs up into a fetal position. I've found that if I straighten the lower leg while keeping the upper bent, then roll forward a bit, I can stretch that hip flexor and lie comfortably balanced. I can even fall asleep in that position.

Messing with your sleep posture is perhaps getting a bit extreme—many people have enough trouble getting to sleep and need very set patterns as it is. But the possible ways you can integrate exercises and better movement patterns into everyday life without carving out more time to schedule them are nearly endless.

Whether better running is worth this level of life integration is up to you. It will require a more mindful focus than many of us are accustomed to. But that focus will also lead to increased skill when you apply it to your running. After these habits and motions have become ingrained, every run works to improve our skill, flexibility, strength, and ability to maintain a more effective stride.

AN INDIVIDUAL JOURNEY

How long will this journey be? Unfortunately, no one can answer that.

First are the questions of where to start and how your body will respond. "You may have a training partner who was a dancer for 30 years. They're going to have more flexibility," says Kastor. That's easier to accept than the second truth, which is that each body has a different response to training stresses. The same exercise, the same stretch, is not going to create the same result in the same time frame for you as it might for the person next door. "The intention has to be to make individual progress," Kastor says. "You're comparing you to you. You should only try to improve upon what you can do."

Not only are our bodies different, but our minds are, too. "Everyone has a different level of kinesthetic awareness, in terms of knowing where their body is in space and how it is moving," says Shultz. Some people can read a description of a plank, for example, and immediately put their body into a perfect position. Others can try the same position and be out of line without knowing it; it requires a photo or video to convince them and hours of work to begin to learn how to feel the spatial positioning and muscles and joints involved.

"Some can get it in a few hours, whereas I have coworkers whom I've been working with for 6 months," Shultz says. "Some people will be frustrated, but it *is* possible. It will just take time."

The end of the journey is to arrive at a place where you sit, stand, and run comfortably and effectively, without having to cue your posture and without pain or performance impediments. Like a line approaching infinity, we may never fully arrive there, particularly if lifestyle patterns fight against us. But we can get to a point where we move better, feel younger, and run faster—by applying the same mind-set we've used to build our running fitness.

Tolstoy said, "The two most powerful warriors are patience and time." As distance runners, we know this is true about fitness and racing prowess. If we want to be better runners, we need to apply these warriors to building our bodies and skills as well.

11
THE MYTH
OF MAGIC SHOES

WHAT A SHOE CAN AND CAN'T DO, AND SOME HELP ON FINDING THE BEST ONES FOR YOU

IN THE CLIMACTIC SCENE OF the 1993 movie *The Sandlot,* just before the athletic hero decides to take on the massive dog by simply outsprinting him, he reveals his "secret weapon: shoes guaranteed to make a kid run faster and jump higher." The shoes in question turned out to be PF Flyers. In the direct-to-DVD 2005 sequel, the shoes are a pair of Nike Cortezes. In both movies, the kid dons the shoes and goes on to be the hero.

Whatever the shoes, the scene highlights the persistent belief that shoes can make you a better athlete. It's a belief nearly all runners have held on to since they were kids. How often have you pored over the *Runner's World* shoe guide, lusting for the pair that would transform you into the runner you know you can be?

Runners aren't alone in this belief that a purchase will make them better: Many middle-aged men think a Porsche will keep them younger and sexier, just as many managers are convinced that the latest tech tool or software will finally get them organized. Advertising thrives on these beliefs and constantly feeds them.

The advertising works because there is a bit of truth there: The right things can improve your looks, your management skills, and more—and the right shoes can make running more comfortable and help you run faster. But shoes, like things in other spheres of life, can only enable what you already have the capacity to do; they cannot, by magic, make you what you are not.

BEWARE THE MYSTICAL BEAST

Making us believe in the myth of magic shoes is where both the traditional running shoe model and the minimalist model have often failed. For years, we were told that if we found the right shoe—one that supported our weaknesses and matched our mechanics—we would stride better, avoid injury, and run faster. Minimalism pointed out the errors of these claims, but it fell for a different brand of magic. The minimalists claimed that simply switching our overbuilt shoes for minimal models would automatically make us change our strides to a better, more natural style, thus helping us to avoid injury and run faster.

"Footwear is this mystical beast that has been given far more credit than it deserves," says Simon Bartold, podiatrist, biomechanics researcher, and consultant for Salomon. "The problem with running has got nothing to do with footwear." Runners get injured, Bartold says, because of repetitive stress. Training overwhelmingly accounts for both injury and running improvement.

That said, everyone agrees that shoes do have a large impact on the runner and the running stride. Which is why, besides the influence of marketing, the myths persist. The question of what shoes can and cannot do and how to find the right ones for you could be the topic of its own book. Here, let's look briefly at what we seem to know now and what is important to pay attention to if you're working to improve your stride.

SHOES CAN'T CORRECT YOU

The driving idea at the center of shoe design and prescription for most of running shoe history has been the belief that overpronation—the foot rotating too far inward—is a sign of a poor stride, a cause of injury, and something the shoe should protect against. The pervasiveness of this idea has culminated in what Bartold calls "pronation-ism." A runner goes to a shoe store or podiatrist and comes home devastated. "Oh my god, I've just been told I'm an overpronator and my world has ended," Bartold jokes—a joke with a bite because it is so close to the truth. I've encountered runners, from ages 12 to 70, who have been told they need motion control and consider it a diagnosis, a lifetime sentence to wearing heavy, stiff, controlling shoes.

Despite this persistent emphasis, neither science nor experience has confirmed the connection between pronation and injury. "I think pronation has been given a very bad rap," Bartold says. "It is just a movement, and it is a normal movement, and it is a very essential movement."

Everyone pronates. Some pronate more than others. We can measure the angle of pronation, Bartold explains, but we don't know how much is too much. "We've had this suggestion that somehow we were able to identify what was overpronation," Bartold says. The truth is that some people pronate quite heavily without any ill effects. "Everybody has an envelope of function— we all work in that envelope. For some people it is very narrow; for some, it is wide."

Benno Nigg, one of the world's most respected biomechanics researchers, now retired, agrees, despite most of a lifetime trying to prove otherwise. "When I got into the field, there was never a question that pronation was a major thing," Nigg says. "The only thing I wanted to do was provide proof that it was a bad thing." Over 50 years of studying shoes and runners, however, he failed to find the direct connection between pronation and injury. "The injuries didn't reduce over the 50 years," Nigg says. "The instances [were] about the same."

In a 2015 article in the *British Journal of Sports Medicine,* Nigg writes, "It is difficult to find supporting evidence that foot pronation (eversion) is a strong predictor of injury." And in his 2010 book, *Biomechanics of Sports Shoes,* Nigg writes, "Pronation is a natural movement of the foot and 'excessive pronation' is a very rare phenomenon. Shoe developers, shoe stores, and medical centers should not be too concerned about 'pronation' and 'overpronation.'"

The first danger comes when runners are put in a heavy, stiff motion-control shoe just because of the extent of their pronation, without concern for whether or not that pronation is stressful to their system. Experts agree that the majority of people do not need the level of support they've been wearing.

"Everyone should be in cushion neutral or below," says podiatrist Rob Conenello. Bartold estimates that serious motion-control shoes are necessary for no more than 1 in 1,000 runners. "Most runners simply don't need that kind of stability," he says. Martyn Shorten, head of the research lab BioMechanica, estimates that only 10 percent of runners need any kind of stability in their shoe at all.

Not only do we not know what level of pronation requires support, but the methods typically used to try to control motion are suspect. "You can't control motion," Bartold states. "Science tells us that you can put all this stuff in a shoe and make it very stiff, with motion control, and if you have a foot that pronates, it will pronate very nicely inside that shoe. The whole concept that you can build a shoe that is going to control pronation is fatally flawed."

Once again, Nigg agrees. "The degree to which a change in shoe construction can affect total foot or ankle joint eversion [inward twisting] is small and not relevant," he says. Nigg goes on to say that these "control" devices are not only ineffective but counterproductive. He returns to the idea that each person's body finds a preferred movement path to minimize effort around its specific parameters.

"If you put people in a shoe, they have a preferred moving path, the path of least resistance, where energy demands are at their lowest," Nigg says. "If you start to fiddle around and control movements, these elements may want to throw you out of your preferred movement paths. That means your muscles work against that, and that costs energy. That's not desirable."

It is easy to accept this analysis if the shoe is messing with our natural gait, like being too stiff to let our toes flex, but our prona-tionism makes us think that controlling excessive inward rolling is necessary. Nigg disagrees. "Let's take a person who is heavily pronated," Nigg says. "If you put that person back into straight alignment, that costs energy. They want to pronate, then their muscles have to do something against that, and that certainly is not advantageous."

As a check against going to the other extreme, Shorten agrees that "most stability features don't work," but he is "not ready to throw out the baby with the bathwater." He explains that while science can't very well measure what is happening within a control shoe—and scientists don't even agree on what exactly pronation or overpronation is—in practice, out on the roads, support shoes work for many people, relieving symptoms and allowing them to run comfortably. A 2016 study by the Luxembourg Institute of Health confirmed that people with pronated feet showed a lower risk of injury while wearing motion-control shoes. "Some people need a [Brooks] Adrenaline," Shorten says. He agrees, however, that probably far fewer need a stability shoe than think they do.

The bottom line is that if we want to run better, either to avoid injury or run faster, we shouldn't look to shoes and think they will make up for stride weaknesses. This type of thinking leads to such fallacies as believing you need more shoe because you're increasing your mileage or training for a marathon—because you'll need more support. Bartold thinks the opposite: "If you're marathon training, you're probably going to lose weight, improve your technique. You're probably going to need less shoe as you go along." If your stride is falling apart due to excessive fatigue from your marathon training, the shoe isn't going to prevent you from getting injured—you need to look instead at your training and timing.

Some might argue that a clunky shoe is a small price to pay for protection. But science and years of experience show that the perceived protection is false. "It's a choice borne out of fear, and the fear is not reality—it is probably the opposite of reality," Bartold says. "At the end of the day, in the sport of running, the less shoe you have is better."

SHOES CAN'T CHANGE YOU

Bartold's assertion is echoed by every expert so often that it starts to sound like a refrain: Run in the least shoe you can wear.

That sounds a lot like minimalism. And no one argues with this part of the minimalist creed. "I want my patients to be in the most minimal shoe they can handle," says Conenello. Bartold maintains: "Minimalism brought us a very important message: Why would you run in more shoe than you absolutely have to?"

Before we get to what was good about minimalism, however, let's explore the area where it overpromised. Many who espoused minimalism believed that if you got rid of the overbuilt shoes and ran barefoot or in very little shoe, you would automatically run better and be injury-free. To be fair, few who actually built those shoes or espoused minimalist ideals taught this, but that was the message that got communicated in the populist forum.

"This is one of the reasons minimalism failed; it was seen as a magic bullet—[something that was] going to have this great change overnight," Bartold says. "That was never going to be sustainable. The human body can't respond that quickly."

Timing was one issue; people rushed into the new shoes and didn't prepare for different stresses or transition gradually. But even more damning was the fact that a lot of people simply don't react and change in response to donning different footwear.

Studies, such as research on short-term adaptations conducted in 2014 at East Carolina University, have repeatedly demonstrated that many runners, probably the majority, will not naturally adapt their stride when they change their shoe. "You can change from a 10-millimeter to a 4-millimeter shoe, for example, and probably only 50 percent of the population will actually change their stride," says Bartold. "There's a fair bit of evidence saying [that] even going barefoot, a number of people won't be able to change how they run. Those things are pretty hardwired."

Nigg ascribes this to the preferred movement path that works against changes to try to maintain its learned, most economical patterns. "If you change shoes, the numbers are that 90 percent of runners don't change," Nigg says. When I told him about my results in experimenting with wearable stride monitors and finding that my metrics stayed fairly consistent in a wide variety of shoes, from racing flats to Hokas, he was not at all surprised. "If you put all these gadgets on, they just show you that you are running in the Jonathan style, and the shoe doesn't make a big difference," he said.

Giving up on the myths that shoes can make up for stride deficiencies or that they can magically modify our strides to be better, where does that leave us? Experts still agree that shoes are important. The wrong shoes can detract from performance and the right shoes can help you run better. Here are four assertions that have fairly universal agreement among experts to help you sort out your shoe selection.

1. Run in the Least Shoe Possible

Experts are unanimous in saying that you want the least-supportive shoe that you can wear for at least two reasons: to let the foot do its job and to maximize efficiency.

Overly supportive shoes weaken feet. This was one of the lessons that led to minimalism, and experts agree that it is valid. We've learned that shoes can create what Edward Tenner, PhD, in *Why Things Bite Back* calls "revenge effects." Tenner defines these effects as "the ironic unintended consequences of mechanical, chemical, biological, and medical ingenuity." Ironic, because the negative consequence is often the very problem the intervention was supposed to help. The revenge effect of shoes is that, in wearing models that are designed to reduce injuries by supporting stride and strength weaknesses, we encourage those weaknesses and have lost the ability to run with our most effective stride, which leads to more injuries.

As we discussed in the foot strength chapter, researchers have found this true in the lab and podiatrists have seen its consequences in their clinics. "Say you have a motion-control shoe that has a high arch support and other things," Nigg says. "Because the high arch support is there, you don't need your foot muscles. That means these muscles deteriorate—they are basically gone. In that sense, the shoe can have an effect on pushing you into a direction you don't want to go."

If we want strong, functional feet, it is clear that we don't want to wear any more support than we need. The caveat here is in that last phrase, "than we need." Something similar is added to all the recommendations for running in the "least shoe" possible. Some add quite a list. "The goal of athletic footwear is to have least amount of shoe possible for you to achieve the most stress-free running you can, to improve your strength, to be comfortable, and to perform the task at hand," Bartold says, adding, "The least amount of shoe to achieve those things for some is going to be quite a bit of shoe."

Finding your level of shoe is the trick, of course. Note that, regardless of the support you need, however, all agree that you don't want weight. Lighter is better. This is one of the few statements scientists will state unequivocally. "If you put a lighter shoe on, and every other feature is the same, running economy will change," says Geoff Gray, PhD in physical therapy and founder of the Heeluxe footwear research lab. "That's just the long lever at the end of our body." Simply put, more weight requires more energy to move.

Companies love to load up the tech in their shoes, showing us visible cushioning systems, plastic support parts, control straps.

"These technologies that are added to the shoe, what they did was add weight, that's all they did—they didn't really help the athlete," says Bartold. "Weight is the great enemy of the athlete. I'm extremely antiweight. It is the single most important feature in a shoe. Why the hell would you put something heavier than you need to on your foot?"

"Wear the least amount of shoe you can get away with," says BioMechanica's Martyn Shorten, echoing the refrain. "Don't get something that has all the extra bells and whistles if you don't need them."

2. What Feels Right *Is* Right

How do you find that line in the sand between "least shoe" and "what you need"? In the past, you'd go to a specialty store, they'd assess your level of pronation, and you'd get your prescribed category. If we "flush motion control down the toilet," as Bartold recommends, and thus eliminate the control categories, what should then be our guide?

Shoe guides and specialty stores can help narrow the list. But beware any that rely too heavily on watching you run and assessing your gait. Podiatrist, runner, and shoe expert Paul Langer says, "You could take 10 physical therapists, 10 podiatrists, and 10 rehab doctors and have them look at a runner on a treadmill, and you'll get 30 different descriptions of what they see and the significance of what they see." What hope does a running store salesperson have, then, no matter how experienced he or she is?

"People are so focused on what happens at the ankle and below," says Ryan Green, who manages a specialty store and is a professor of kinesiology. "And running is everything, absolutely everything. You have to look at the whole person."

Shoe fitters should be guiding you to families of shoes, loose groupings with similar characteristics, based on larger categories of information they gather about you. Bartold lists some of these: "gender, body weight, level of expertise, mileage, technique, biomechanics." Good stores do this. Victor Ornelas, senior franchise support manager for Fleet Feet, says they instruct their shoe fitters to interview customers in order to understand their "age, history, fitness levels, goals" before looking at things like foot shape. The *Runner's World* shoe guide directs people to different groupings of shoes based on body mass, running experience, and proneness to injury.

Whether or not you have someone help you narrow the field, in the end, the best sort is going to be finding what works for you. That sounds obvious, but it's the best science offers now, and it's backed by research. Studies by Nigg's group at the University of Calgary have shown that when runners select shoes or inserts they deem the most comfortable, they run more efficiently and have fewer injuries.

These studies have led Nigg to propose the "comfort filter" as the best method for choosing shoes. He ties this to his concept of the preferred movement path: Your body is going to move a certain way—the right shoe will let it move that way without resistance, thus requiring the least muscular action, and thus feeling best. While even Nigg calls the idea a proposal that needs more research, no one has a better plan and experts across the spectrum agree in principle. "The shoe that's going to work best for the athlete is the one that feels the best—that makes complete sense," says Bartold. "Every aspect of the way we move is controlled by the brain, and the brain is a very sophisticated monitoring device."

Note that neither the concept of "preferred movement path"

nor the "comfort filter" eliminates shoes that offer support. Some people will feel most comfortable in a more supportive shoe. Carson Caprara, Brooks's senior footwear product line manager, sees the support as helping your body maintain your natural pattern when your muscles are weak or fatigued. "The support of the shoe, instead of stopping motion, is supporting the preferred motion," Caprara explains.

Whether or not an element like a medial post, a firmer material under the arch side of the foot, actually controls pronation is irrelevant if it creates a feeling that works for you. It may simply create a more solid base. "[Our view is that] medial posting and control features built into stability shoes are designed more to prolong the shoe as a neutral platform, not to alter control of the foot—[they're] more of a durability component of the shoe," says Fleet Feet's Ornelas. Luke Rowe, vice president of business development for Fleet Feet, echoes this: "Think about it as how much durability does the customer need? The biomechanics may be the same, but the type of footwear a runner needs to wear at 200 pounds is far different than one at 140 pounds."

Regardless of what specific features a shoe has, your foot's perception of a shoe's comfort encompasses the whole shoe—the shape, the angle of impact, the density of materials, the upper—all of which affect stability, cushioning, and ride. When you let your body assess what feels right, it frees you from the prison of shoe categories and the trap of relying on one factor such as whether or not the shoe has a medial post.

FINDING COMFORT

Biomechanics researcher Jay Dicharry agrees with Nigg's ideas on preferred movement paths but has concerns over whether runners can use comfort in a convenient way to select shoes. "A lot of runners don't try enough different shoes," Dicharry says. "They've been in the same shoe for a long time, and they're not willing to try something slightly different, let alone radically different."

Dicharry also fears that an emphasis on comfort, as generally understood, encourages the perception that more is always better, and that a squishy marshmallow foam that feels good while walking around a store will be deemed appropriate for one's tempo runs.

Rather than the term "comfort," Geoff Gray likes to describe it as, "the product that moves with your body well." In his experience watching thousands of runners test and evaluate shoes, he says, "For most people, comfort is just cushion—and usually cushion they feel in the first 10 seconds. That is so influencing to people."

That 10-second cushion feel is not the assessment Nigg intends, either. "There's a difference between short-term comfort and long-term comfort," he says. "The short-term comfort is probably how you buy the shoe. You shouldn't just slip into the shoe and say, 'that's nice.' You should take them out and run around a little bit, then you feel the long-term comfort."

When a shoe is right, the feeling is of things falling into place: You land where you expect to land, the shoe bends where it is supposed to bend, you push off smoothly and powerfully, the cushioning is the right density to feel good but not swallow or slow your stride, and the support is invisible, not too much or too little. You may not be able to identify all these features, but if it feels smooth and right—it all works.

Even accepting this definition, Shorten has concerns with the fact that comfort is a psychological outcome, not a characteristic of a shoe, and as such it makes it difficult to measure accurately. "The sensation of comfort is imperfect and not very repeatable,"

Shorten says. "On a given day, it is biased by each subject's experience, their mood, the environment, and many other factors."

Even Nigg and his team admit to observing difficulties in the ability to assess comfort accurately. Sandro Nigg, Benno's son and the owner of Biomechanigg Sport and Health Research, points to a 2002 study conducted by their group that showed that two-thirds of the subjects struggled to provide a consistent assessment of the comfort of shoe inserts on a sliding scale from day to day. They were more consistent with a simple "Yes/No" response to "Is this insert comfortable?" but still had less than 50 percent consistency.

How best to counteract this? First, make sure you try on multiple shoes. It is easier to compare comfort between shoes than to assign a value to one. "You may try on one pair and think, 'These are pretty good,'" Sandro Nigg says. "But then you try on another and find they are better."

Next, don't get locked into a certain category or brand: Try shoes from a wide spectrum. At the very least, there may be a lower threshold of comfort, Sandro Nigg suggests. "You can tell when something is uncomfortable, and you can stay away from those 'bad' shoes for you."

Dicharry adds: "If you're going to use the shoe for fast running, run fast in it. When speed changes, your stride changes, and how the shoe behaves changes." Taking the shoes through multiple paces gives your body more chances to identify elements of the shoe that might detract. Good specialty stores should allow this kind of test drive.

For those who have a poor or inconsistent sense of comfort, who buy shoes that feel right in the store then find they often don't work on the road, Sandro Nigg says first get help assessing characteristics of your body and running experience, as described above, to narrow your selection to ones that are the most likely to work for you. "Then you try them on and the comfort is the validation: 'yes, this is comfortable,'" Nigg says.

3. Fit Matters More Than Features

While the "comfort filter" covers the performance of the shoe, it also applies to fit. And fit, while often overlooked in our fascination with midsoles, might be even more important when it comes to how a shoe affects your stride.

"Fit dramatically changes how you interact with the shoe," says Gray. "And if you change how you interact with the shoe, that's going to change how you run. The shoe should accentuate your ability to interact with the ground, not limit it."

The biggest error people make is in shoe size. Gray tests runners every day, including assessing how their feet move inside shoes. "We have something like 320 people in our database," he says. "Of those people, three-quarters of them are coming in a half size smaller than they should be."

The problem with shoes that are too small is that they limit the ability of your foot to flex and splay, both of which are critical to an effective stride. If your shoe is too short or too narrow, for example, it will affect your pushoff. "If there is some pinching on the toes, and you have good hip extension and you're getting good flex through the toes, your body recognizes that that is when the toes are getting squeezed the most," Gray says. "It is uncomfortable, so you'll start shortening up your stride or you'll start to push off with more pronation. Your body will make these micro-adjustments to get rid of that sensation. Your body is going to create limits somewhere so you don't get there."

Gray sees several critical areas for fit.

- **LENGTH.** "Your toes are supposed to be a thumbs-width away from the end of the shoe—that's important, because when you flex the shoe, as it bends, your toes are going to get closer to the edge."

- **TOP OF THE FOOT, THE INSTEP.** "Laces need to lock down on that area and give a secure fit. If you're not secure there, nothing else matters: It's going to be impossible to get a good-fitting running shoe."

- **HEEL.** "You want a secure fit to prevent the foot sliding up and down while pushing off, and you also don't want sliding side to side."

- **BALL OF FOOT.** Make sure it is wide enough. "The easiest way to determine if the shoe fits well: if you can actively spread your toes out and bring them back together as far as you would if you weren't inside of a shoe."

Natural running expert Mark Cucuzzella, MD, agrees with the emphasis on length and width: He reminds us that your foot under load will lengthen by up to half an inch and will splay by 15 percent—if allowed by the shoe. Get up on your ball in the shoe, put weight on it, and make it flex. Make sure the shoe is not restricting this movement.

END TOE MAIMING

This last item of fit is perhaps the most important, and the hardest to find. The idea that shoes need to be wide enough in the forefoot to allow the foot to splay somehow got thrown out with the rest of the minimalist/barefoot movement. But podiatrists, physical therapists, and those who research feet say that crimping the forefoot doesn't allow the foot to operate properly.

What is more, if the toebox is narrower than the ball of the foot, you are deforming your feet. "More than half of the people in the United States have foot deformity as a result of wearing shoes," says Shorten. "People end up with the shape of the toes looking like the shape of a running shoe." And it isn't supposed to look that way.

"Your foot is widest at the toes—but most shoes aren't built that way," says Cucuzzella. As a result of this shape, podiatrist Ray McClanahan says, "If you're an active adult American, you are slowly maiming your feet—and by extension, the rest of your body." He points out that bunions don't exist where people don't wear constrictive shoes. A bunion, in fact, is not a bone issue but "a progressive dislocation of the big toe joint."

The implications of this dislocation are significant. When your toe is pushing inward, you can't form your arch properly, and you lose foot strength and balance as a result. This then leads to problems up the chain, in the knee and hip. "If you can't stabilize your foot, you can't prepare for propulsion," McClanahan says. "Your brain senses that, and it is not going to let other prime movers do their jobs, because it realizes the foundation is not stable enough to do that."

McClanahan has devised a plastic insert, Correct Toes, that helps push your toes back to a natural splay, and he agrees that all the foot exercises are helpful. But he feels the most important step to correct your feet is to get shoes that don't perpetuate the problem. "If you're going to wear a shoe for 8 hours with your toes pinched in, I don't know how much good you're going to do [with] 10 to 15 minutes a day doing rehab on your foot," he says. "It has everything to do with periodically kicking your shoes off, and, when you're not barefoot, try[ing] to be in a shoe that lets you spread your toes out a little bit."

Shoes across the board are starting to improve in this aspect, but nearly all are still narrower at the toe. It looks right to us, and companies cater to fashion. A few companies, notably Altra and Topo, and several minimalist shoe companies, treat this seriously and build shoes with room for your toes to align as they did when you were born. If you're serious about letting your feet move naturally, they are worth trying, even if people consider them "clown shoes." If nothing else, take width seriously and get shoes that let your toes move.

4. Shoe Monogamy Is Not a Virtue

As with training, variety is not only the spice of life but also essential to optimizing the stresses of shoes and your stride. Every time you put on a different pair of shoes, your interaction with the ground changes slightly. "It's a two-way highway," says Gray. "What are we feeling and perceiving, and what are we able to put onto the ground. Shoes affect both pathways."

A 2012 study by the Sports Medicine Research Laboratory in Luxembourg showed that those who ran in a variety of footwear had fewer injuries. It is one of the easiest elements to manipulate, and each shoe presents the body with a different set of stresses, as well as different parameters, encouraging rewiring—particularly after gaining new strengths and mobility.

In the case of shoes, too many runners are monogamous. Once they've experimented with several models, many runners find one shoe they like and state their lifelong loyalty. They then run in the same shoe every day, replace them with the same model, and even stockpile them for the coming apocalypse of discontinuation.

While you may argue this fits with the preferred movement path and comfort models, it also leads to the plasticity ruts we want to avoid. A healthy runner should have a variety of possible patterns. "There is no best footwear," says Bartold, who encourages runners to have different shoes for different runs. "If you want to go faster, you probably want something lighter, with less drop."

Play the field with shoes. You can have different shoes at the same time: a different pair for speed work than for long runs, for example. Maybe another pair for recovery days when you're feeling beat up. A pair for off-road running. And you certainly want to change consecutively—try a different pair when you replace your shoes.

YOU'VE CHANGED, SO SHOULD YOUR SHOES

One key reason to start fresh every time you replace your shoes is that your needs and preferences can have changed. Benno Nigg makes it clear that preferred movement patterns are relative to the body you have at the moment. If you change that body, your movements will change and your shoe preferences will change. If you're doing the posture, mobility, glute, and core work recommended in this book, and your stride is getting more efficient, you're likely going to want a different shoe.

"Once you move differently, you're going to need less shoe," says Bartold. The improved runner finds, "Now, I'm more functionally efficient, I'm functionally strong, I've lost weight, I've improved my technique so I'm not overstriding, so I don't need massive amounts of rearfoot cushioning or support—so I can operate with much less shoe."

Nigg says that the comfort filter will identify what you need now, not an ideal version of you or the person you were last year. "It supports what you have at the moment," he says. What you have is going to be influenced by what your body has adapted to, so be careful with huge changes. Your shoes, however, can and should change if your body and habits change.

Don't fall into the trap that only one shoe is going to work for you and nothing could ever compare. Models change over time. Your perfect shoe may have subtle, or not so subtle, modifications that change how it responds and moves with your foot. Alternatively, I've encountered many runners who, having had a bad experience with one shoe, dismiss not only the model but the brand forever. But companies release new models with new materials and designs every season.

Even if you love your current shoe, it is worth looking around. "Product testers come in and find what works for them best," says Gray. "But then [they might] try something else and say, 'This is even better!' It is good to be open that something can be even better than you are used to."

DAILY SHOES

One final thought on shoes, which is stressed by every podiatrist: Be mindful of the shoes you wear every day. First, make sure they have room for your toes, both in length and width.

Casual shoes are also a good place to experiment with a lower heel-toe drop. "You don't hear of people getting walking injuries," says Cucuzzella. Even if you run in a shoe with a higher heel—because that is what you're used to and feels best to you—a lower-drop, more minimal casual shoe will introduce variety, stretch your Achilles, encourage foot strength, and invite a landing closer beneath your body. Fortunately, more shoe companies are making workday shoes that are attractive as well as functional. Check out options by Altra, Lems, Vivobarefoot, and Xero.

12
FORM CUES

A FEW THINGS TO THINK ABOUT ON THE RUN

OFTEN, WHEN PEOPLE THINK OF better form, they look for cues to change their patterns or to remind them to stride a certain way. But many cues are difficult to implement or can create unnatural patterns, which can lead to injury. Trying to land on your forefoot or midfoot, trying to decrease your ground contact time, trying to change your stride length or pronate less—all are nearly impossible to do simply by thinking about them. If you do manage to change, often it will mess with your mechanics and preferred movement patterns. Other cues are simply too general and hard to follow, such as "use your arms," or "stride out."

A few cues seem to be universally accepted among coaches, scientists, and sports-med professionals. These seem simple, perhaps too simple. But that is their beauty: They are simple enough to perform correctly and, when implemented, create changes that enhance but do not alter your form. Following is a short list of cues I've found helpful.

RUN TALL

On a track nestled in the mountains of eastern California, I watched coach Andrew Kastor conducting a morning speed workout for the Mammoth Track Club, which includes both international elites and community road runners. As the intervals took their toll and the runners started to tire, Kastor implored them to "Run tall!" If there is one cue that stands above all advice on running better, this is it.

Good coaches universally agree. Greg McMillan wrote a Performance Page training column in *Running Times* on running tall, calling it, "the simplest, most effective running form cue" and claiming that it "will clear up about 90 percent of form issues."

Coach G. P. Pearlberg wrote a book centered on the idea: *Run Tall, Run Easy.* "Whether you are on a neighborhood jog or a peak-season race, the taller you are relative to your own height, the better your running will be," Pearlberg wrote.

Running tall simply means being as upright and balanced as possible. As we've talked about elsewhere, it starts with the hips. To get tall, you need to pull your butt in, rotate your hips back, straighten your spine, and lift your chest up. Moving up, your shoulders are back and above your spine. Your head is over your shoulders and high on your straight neck. Many suggest imagining a line attached to the top of your head, pulling you upward.

You needn't be tall to run tall. I've heard petite women joke multiple times, "What if I'm not tall?" Like everything else, tall is relative—it's about getting as tall as you can, feeling tall, thinking tall.

A proper forward lean also does not change running tall.

You're still upright from heel to head, with the balance simply shifted slightly forward. Think of the line attached to your head lifting and gently pulling forward at the same time.

When fatigue starts to compromise your form, thinking "tall" is the simplest, most effective cue to stay balanced and running efficiently and effectively.

ELBOWS BACK

After running tall, the second most universally agreed-upon cue I've discovered is to drive your arms back. Kastor says the one thing he typically yells in a race, where the runner can only hear and implement something simple, is, "elbows back." Physical therapist Abby Douek cues runners to touch their waistband with each stride, ensuring that the arm is driving back and opening up behind the body.

When you drive your elbows back, it cues the legs to drive backward. This is particularly key later in a race when you tend to lose power. Drive your arms and your legs will follow.

Driving your arms backward also shifts your balance more upright and forward (run tall!) so that your feet can land closer beneath your body and push backward. Keeping your arms back can do more for your foot strike than thinking about where your feet are landing.

Keeping your arms back also helps ensure that your movement and force all travel in a forward and backward direction. Besides throwing off your front-to-rear balance, if your arms stay in front of your body, they'll tend to travel back and forth across the midline, misdirecting motion and wasting force in sideways and rotational movements.

RUN SOFT, RUN QUIET

This cue has scientific backing: In a 2010 controlled study by Harrison Crowell and Irene Davis at the University of Delaware's Motion Analysis Laboratory, runners who were told to run softly and more quietly were able to reduce their foot impact and, after six sessions, retained the change for at least a month. In the study, the runners also had the benefit of being able to see a visual display of their impact for immediate feedback, which was gradually removed as the study progressed. Not having access to visual impact feedback, you'll have to rely on the sound of your footsteps and the internal feelings of impact. Which, it seems from my experience, can be enough.

Other coaches confirm what I have seen, that runners are able to run more smoothly simply by trying to make less noise. This works in combination with running tall, keeping your elbows back, and striding quickly to cue a light, dancing stride. Coach Bobby McGee says, "Avoid muscling the run. Think about running on thin ice." He can tell when a runner is getting better because her stride is quieter and he can't pick her out from among a group. "Learn that proprioceptive control equals quietness," he says. "Smooth, light, quiet, compact."

CLIMBING HARNESS

This cue I have adapted from various sources, and it tends to help with posture and lightness in your stride. It goes along with running tall, but, since it is a bit more complex, is rarely yelled from the sidelines. I explain it in workouts to use as a visual, imaginary aid during runs.

Imagine that you have a climbing harness on, such as used for a zip line or rappelling. It wraps around your waist and each leg and has a clip in front beneath your belly button. Attached to that clip is a line that pulls up and forward. (Former Olympian, author, and coach Lorraine Moller suggests that you imagine that it is attached to a hot-air balloon being blown forward in front of you.)

The tension on the line keeps your hips forward and posture tall, avoiding the "sitting" position. It also cues a light landing as the harness holds you up, letting your feet drive and push off beneath and behind.

Another cue that produces a similar feeling is to imagine a hand on your lower back, just at the base of your spine, gently pushing you forward.

SKATEBOARD

A cue I've heard from Coaches Grant Robison and Tom Miller and the experts at Lumo Bodytech is to think about being on a skateboard or scooter (Miller actually recommends getting an adult-sized scooter). The key in the visualization is that on a skateboard you never land in front and brake, but instead you bring your leg through in a swinging motion, touching down beneath you and then driving straight back. If you do the same when running, you'll cue a landing closer to the body in front, a long stride out the back—using your glutes—and a straight push back, not rotating inward. All of these are keys to a powerful, effective stride.

MIDRUN STRIDERS

One of the most counterintuitive cues to shake up your stride midrun is to speed up when you feel tired. A high school state cross-country champion I coached, Scott Ohlson, used to claim to do this, causing raised eyebrows and eye rolling around the team when he talked about it. But Douek recommends it as well and explains why it works. "Distance runners often fall into old patterns when they are fatigued or think they need to go slowly to do more mileage," Douek says. She teaches people instead to speed up for 10-second bursts every 5 to 7 minutes of the run after the onset of sluggish fatigue feelings. You don't want to sprint, just to pick up the cadence and the speed slightly. It can make it feel easier and more natural, even though you are going faster.

"You can change those muscle groups—get out of your hip flexors, into your glutes," Douek says. "When you are tired, that's when I want you to add a stride in, because you've sat back into the wrong muscles again. It is completely counterintuitive, you think you are tired, you've got to slow down. But no, I actually want you to turn it up a notch." Once you change the muscle groups you are using, focus on holding that form as you return to your slower, longer-run speed.

THE HALLELUJAH DRILL

A cue I've heard from several experts including Max King, Grant Robison, and Golden Harper—all elite runners and coaches—is to reach for the sky while on the run. We've talked about reaching high to cue standing tall and to get your hips in line in the context of a posture assessment or before drills or starting a run. This is similar, but instead you do it in full stride.

When you feel yourself starting to sag and slouch in the middle or late miles of a run, straighten up and throw your arms up high, then let the momentum swing them around in a big circle and back up into your running position by your sides. You'll find that your posture is now taller, your chest is high, your shoulders and arms are back, and there is a smile on your face. You don't have to yell "Hallelujah!" when you do this.

"Lifting your hands over head while running doesn't do as much as when you're standing still," Robison says. "But [it] makes you aware and gets you [away] from being hunched over. Most people, when they get tired, are going to sit into their stride, drift backward. Putting your arms over your head reminds you to get tall. Tall and light." In the end, that is the goal: to get tall and light.

13
ACTION PLAN

A QUICK OVERVIEW OF THE STEPS TO START STRIDING BETTER

THE PREVIOUS CHAPTERS TOOK US through the science and necessary work toward a better stride. Here is a quick overview to know where you're going and spur you to start now.

- ❯ **ADD SPICE.** Mix up your training paces, terrain, and shoes. The first step to running better is to let your body optimize itself. To do so, it needs to break out of ruts and be given options. If you do nothing else, you will be a better runner if you do this: Run often. At different paces. Mostly easy.

- ❯ **GET INSPIRED.** Watch videos of elite athletes like Kenenisa Bekele, Tirunesh Dibaba, Shalane Flanagan, Meb Keflezighi, and Galen Rupp. Pay attention to their posture, their hips, and the way the tops of their legs move.

- ❯ **SHIFT YOUR STRIDE.** Work toward moving the power stroke of your stride behind you so that you push, not pull. To do this, work on these four areas.

  1. **Get tall.** Assess your hip posture and start learning a new neutral balance.

2. **Make sure you can move.** Assess your hip extension and start stretching to improve your range of motion.

3. **Build a better butt.** Get your glutes activated and start strengthening them.

4. **Bring your arms back.** Get your shoulders and arms back through stretching, mobilization, and cuing.

❭ **SHORE UP THE FOUNDATION.** Improve your foot strength, mobility, and proprioception to improve your balance, pop off the ground faster, and reduce injury risk.

❭ **STEP QUICKLY.** Play with different cadences to find your optimal ranges at different speeds and to mix up how you move so that your body integrates new abilities.

❭ **MIX IT UP MORE.** Add drills to improve your range of motion and to recruit new muscles and patterns. Get off-road: Sprint down a mountain or up a hill. Get barefoot. Play Frisbee. Try a different brand and style of shoe. Push yourself a few times per week. Do intervals on grass. Give your body a chance to find and adopt better ways of moving.

❭ **GET REAL.** Integrate posture, mobility, and strength work into your daily life to reinforce new habits and build the postural endurance necessary to stay tall and balanced during all of your runs.

❭ **BE A CHILD.** In actions and attitude, be open to the new, physically and intellectually. It's harder to make changes after age 30—so don't act your age. Relearn how to play. Don't be afraid to look and act goofy. Let people see you sweat, get out of your comfort zone, be willing to fail. Keep learning. Be open to new ideas, even those that contradict what you think you know.

ACKNOWLEDGMENTS

THE BEST PART ABOUT WRITING a book is the chance to talk at length with brilliant people about something I'm interested in. I'm grateful for the time and expertise shared with me by Simon Bartold, Laura Bergmann, Markus Blomqvist, Rob Conenello, Brad Cox, Mark Cucuzzella, Irene Davis, Jay Dicharry, Abby Douek, Brian Fullem, Jeff Gaudette, Geoffrey Gray, Ryan Green, Brian Heiderscheit, Andrew Kastor, John Kiely, Paul Langer, Daniel Lieberman, Ray McClanahan, Bobby McGee, David McHenry, Jordan Metzl, Tom Miller, Trent Nessler, Grant Robison, Benno Nigg, Sandro Nigg, Martyn Shorten, Scott Simmons, Rebecca Shultz, Lee Troop, Phil Wharton, and many others.

Thanks goes to Coach Carl Zuege and the Chase County cross-country team for being my daily test subjects and reality check.

The *Running Times* staff, including Scott Douglas, Sarah Lorge Butler, Brian Metzler, Erin Strout, and Renee Bottom, encouraged me to pursue this idea and edited the first version that appeared as a feature story in that magazine.

Mark Weinstein, my editor at Rodale, carefully corrected my copy, tightened my thinking and my prose, and encouraged me with his positive reactions to my ideas. Nancy N. Bailey and Jo Ann Learman further refined both the accuracy and clarity of the text.

I appreciate *Runner's World* editors David Willey and John Atwood for their support of this project from beginning to end.

Finally, my largest thanks goes to my wife, Tracy, who patiently lived with me carrying around 50,000 words in my head for several months while providing the time and encouragement for me to get them in the right order. She also compiled a mess of links and a stack of books and papers into a bibliography.

BIBLIOGRAPHY

BOOKS

Abshire, Danny, with Brian Metzler. *Natural Running: The Simple Path to Stronger, Healthier Running.* Boulder, CO: VeloPress, 2010.

Anderson, Owen. *Running Science: The Ultimate Nexus of Knowledge and Performance.* Champaign, IL: Human Kinetics, 2013.

Cavanagh, Peter R. *The Running Shoe Book.* Mountain View, CA: Anderson World, Inc., 1980.

Culpepper, Alan, with Brian Metzler. *Run Like a Champion: An Olympian's Approach for Every Runner.* Boulder, CO: VeloPress, 2015.

Daniels, Jack. *Daniels' Running Formula.* Champaign, IL: Human Kinetics, 1998.

Dicharry, Jay. *Anatomy for Runners: Unlocking Your Athletic Potential for Health, Speed, and Injury Prevention.* New York: Skyhorse Publishing, 2012.

Douglas, Scott. *The Runner's World Complete Guide to Minimalism and Barefoot Running: How to Make the Healthy Transition to Lightweight Shoes and Injury-Free Running.* Emmaus, PA: Rodale, 2013.

Dreyer, Danny, and Katherine Dreyer. *Chi Running: A Revolutionary Approach to Effortless, Injury-Free Running.* New York: Simon & Schuster, 2004.

Glover, Bob, and Shelly-Lynn Florence Glover. *The Competitive Runner's Handbook.* New York: Penguin Books, 1999.

Glover, Bob, Jack Shepherd, and Shelly-Lynn Florence Glover. *The Runner's Handbook.* New York: Penguin Books, 1996.

Keflezighi, Meb, with Douglas Scott. *Meb for Mortals; How to Run, Think, and Eat Like a Champion Marathoner.* Emmaus, PA: Rodale, 2015.

Larson, Peter, and Bill Katovsky. *Tread Lightly: Form, Footwear, and the Quest for Injury-Free Running.* New York: Skyhorse Publishing, 2012.

Lieberman, Daniel. *The Story of the Human Body; Evolution, Health, and Disease.* New York: Vintage Books, a Division of Random House, 2014.

Magill, Pete, Thomas Schwartz, and Melissa Breyer. *Build Your Running Body: A Total-Body Fitness Plan for All Distance Runners from Milers to Ultramarathoners.* New York: The Experiment, 2014.

Martin, Brian. *Running Technique.* Published by Brian Martin, 2011.

Metzl, Jordan D. *Dr. Jordan Metzl's Running Strong: The Sports Doctor's Complete Guide to Staying Healthy and Injury-Free for Life.* Emmaus, PA: Rodale, 2015.

Miller, Thomas S. *Programmed to Run: Develop Elite Running/Racing Biomechanical and Mental Skills, Regardless of Age, Gender, or Body Type.* Champaign, IL: Human Kinetics, 2002.

Nigg, Benno M. *Biomechanics of Sports Shoes.* Calgary, Alberta, Can.: University of Calgary, 2010.

Pearlberg, G. P. *Run Tall, Run Easy: The Ultimate Guide to Better Running Mechanics.* Champaign, IL: 42K + Press, 2008.

Pirie, Gordon. *Running Fast and Injury Free.* UK: John S. Gilbody, 2004.

Romanov, Nicholas, with John Robson. *Pose Method of Running: A New Paradigm of Running.* Coral Gables, FL: PoseTech Press, 2002.

Starrett, Kelly, and T. J. Murphy. *Ready to Run: Unlocking Your Potential to Run Naturally.* Las Vegas, NV: Victory Belt Publishing, 2014.

Tenner, Edward. *Why Things Bite Back: Technology and the Revenge of Unintended Consequences.* New York: Knopf, 1996.

Vance, Jim. *Run with Power: the Complete Guide to Power Meters for Running.* Boulder, CO: VeloPress, 2016.

Wharton, Jim, and Phil Wharton. *The Whartons' Back Book: End Back Pain—Now and Forever—with This Simple, Revolutionary Program.* Emmaus, PA: Rodale, 2003.

PROFESSIONAL JOURNAL ARTICLES AND PRESENTATIONS

Bartold, Simon. "Biomechanics of Running Shoes." Presented at the American Association of Podiatric Sports Medicine's Stand-Alone Meeting, West Point, New York. September 11, 2015.

Bontekoning, I. Y. "Plea for the Free Foot, A Different Perspective on Feet." *De Medische Voet (The Medical Foot),* February 2014.

———. "Strong and Intrinsic Foot Muscles Prevent and Correct Foot Complaints." *De Medische Voet (The Medical Foot),* April 2015.

Cavanagh, Peter R., and Keith R. Williams. "The Effect of Stride Length Variation on Oxygen Uptake During Distance Running." *Medicine and Science in Sports and Exercise* 14, no. 1 (1982): 30–35.

Conenello, Robert. "Dynamic Assessment." Presented at The Running Event conference, Austin, Texas, December 5, 2013.

Cox, Bradley. "The Missing Link for Running Efficiency: Upper Body Mechanics." Presented at the American Medical Association's 45th Annual Sports Medicine Symposium at the Boston Marathon, April 16, 2016.

Crowell, Harrison P., and Irene S. Davis. "Gait Retraining to Reduce Lower Extremity Loading in Runners." *Clinical Biomechanics* 26, no. 1 (January 2011): 78–83.

Cucuzzella, Mark. "Gait as Rehab." Presented at the American Association of Podiatric Sports Medicine's Stand Alone Meeting, United States Military Academy, West Point, New York. September 11, 2015. http://www.usafp.org/wp-content/uploads/2016/03/Cucuzzella-Running.pdf.

Daoud, Adam I., et al. "Foot Strike and Injury Rates in Endurance Runners: A Retrospective Study." *Medicine and Science in Sports Exercise* 44, no. 7 (July 2012):1325–34. doi: 10.1249/MSS.0b013e3182465115.

David, Irene S., et al. "Greater Vertical Impact Loading in Female Runners with Medically Diagnosed Injuries: A Prospective Investigation." *British Journal of Sports Medicine* 50, no. 14 (July 2016): 887–92. doi: 10.1136/bjsports-2015-094579.

De Ruiter, Cornelis J., et al. "Stride Frequency in Relation to Oxygen Consumption in Experienced and Novice Runners." *European Journal of Sport Science* 14, no. 3 (2014): 251–58. doi: 10.1080/17461391.2013.783627.

Dicharry, Jay M., et al. "Differences in Static and Dynamic Measures in Evaluation of Talonavicular Mobility in Gait." *Journal of Orthopaedic and Sports Physical Therapy* 39, no. 8 (August 2009): 628–34. doi: 10.2519/jospt.2009.2968.

Ferber, Reed, et al. "Competitive Female Runners with a History of Iliotibial Band Syndrome Demonstrate Atypical Hip and Knee Kinematics." *Journal of Orthopaedic and Sports Physical Therapy* 40, no. 2 (February 2010): 52–58.

Fredericson, M., et al. "Hip Abductor Weakness in Distance Runners with Iliotibial Band Syndrome." *Clinical Journal of Sports Medicine* 10, no. 3 (July 2000): 169–75.

Gallam, George M., et al. "Effect of a Global Alteration of Running Technique on Kinematics and Economy." *Journal of Sports Sciences* 23, no. 7 (2005 Jul): 757–64.

Glasoe, Ward M. "Treatment of Progressive First MTP Hallux Valgus Deformity: A Biomechanically-Based Muscle Strengthening Approach." *Journal of Orthopaedic & Sports Physical Therapy* 46, no. 7 (2016): 596–605. doi: 10.2519 /jospt.2016.6704.

Gordon, Joshua P. "High Resolution MEMS Accelerometers to Compare Running Mechanics between Trained and Untrained Runners." *Medicine & Science in Sports & Exercise* 42, no. 5 (May 2010). doi: 10.1249/01. mss.0000385947.02061.c6.

Goss, Donald L., et al. "Lower Extremity Biomechanics and Self-Reported Foot-Strike Patterns Among Runners in Traditional and Minimalist Shoes." *Journal of Athletic Training* 50, no. 6 (June 2015): 603–11. doi: 10.4085/1062-6050-49.6.06.

Gruber, Allison H., et al. "Economy and Rate of Carbohydrate Oxidation During Running with Rearfoot and Forefoot Strike Patterns." *Journal of Applied Physiology* 115, no. 2 (May 2013): 194–201. doi: 10.1152/japplphysiol.01437.2012.

Hafer, Jocelyn F., et al. "The Effect of a Cadence Retraining Protocol on Running Biomechanics and Efficiency: A Pilot Study." *Journal of Sports Sciences* 33, no. 7 (2015): 724–31.

Hamill, Joseph, Christopher Palmer, and Richard E. A. Van Emmerik. "Coordinative Variability and Overuse Injury." *Sports Medicine, Arthroscopy, Rehabilitation, Therapy & Technology* 45, no. 4 (2012). doi: 10.1186/1758-2555-4-45.

Hamill, Joseph, et al. "A Dynamical Systems Approach to Lower Extremity Running Injuries." *Clinical Biomechanics* 14, no. 5 (June 1999): 297–308.

Hasegawa, Hiroshi, Takeshi Yamauchi, and William J. Kraemer. "Foot Strike Patterns of Runners at the 15-Km Point During an Elite-Level Half Marathon." *Journal of Strength & Conditioning Research* 21, no. 3 (August 2007): 888–93.

Hatala, Kevin G., et al. "Variation in Foot Strike Patterns During Running among Habitually Barefoot Populations." *PLoS ONE* 8, no. 1 (2013): e52548. doi: 10.1371/journal.pone.0052548.

Heiderscheit, Bryan C. "Running Form Modification: When Self-Selected Is Not Preferred." Proceedings, American Physical Therapy Association Combined Sections Meeting, San Diego, CA, February 7, 2010.

Heiderscheit, Bryan C., et al. "Effects of Step Rate Manipulation on Joint Mechanics during Running." *Medicine and Science in Sports and Exercise* 43, no. 2 (February 2011): 296–302. doi: 10.1249/MSS.0b013e3181ebedf4m.

Kasmer, Mark E., et al. "Foot-Strike Pattern and Performance in a Marathon." *International Journal of Sports Physiological Performance* 8, no. 3 (2013 May): 286–92.

Keller, Tony S., et al. "Relationship Between Vertical Ground Reaction Force and Speed During Walking, Slow Jogging, and Running." *Clinical Biomechanics* 11, no. 5 (July 1996): 253–59.

Kerrigan, D. Casey, et al. "The Effect of Running Shoes on Lower Extremity Joint Torques." *PM&R* 1, no. 12 (December 2009): 1058–63. http://dx.doi.org/10.1016/j.pmrj.2009.09.011.

Kiely, John. "Running Coordination: The Purpose of Coordination." Prepublication excerpt courtesy of author, 2016.

Kim, Moon-Hwan, et al. "Effect of Toe-Spread-Out Exercise on Hallux Valgus Angle and Cross-Sectional Area of Abductor Hallucis Muscle in Subjects with Hallux Valgus." *Journal of Physical Therapy Science* 27, no. 4 (April 2015): 1019–22. doi: 10.1589/jpts.27.1019.

Kirby, Kevin A. "Emerging Evidence on Foot-Strike Patterns in Running." *Podiatry Today* 27, no. 6 (June 2014). http://www.podiatrytoday.com/emerging-evidence-footstrike-patterns-running.

Lack, Simon, et al. "Proximal Muscle Rehabilitation Is Effective for Patellofemoral Pain: A Systematic Review with Meta-Analysis." *British Journal of Sports Medicine* 49, no. 21 (2015): 1365–76. doi: 10.1136/bjsports-2015-094723.

Lieberman, Daniel E., et al. "Effects of Stride Frequency and Foot Position at Landing on Braking Force, Hip Torque, Impact Peak Force, and the Metabolic Cost of Running in Humans." *Journal of Experimental Biology* 218, no. 21 (2015): 3406–14. doi: 10.1242/jeb.125500.

Lenhart, Rachel, et al. "Hip Muscle Loads During Running at Various Step Rates." *Journal of Orthopaedic & Sports Physical Therapy* 44, no. 10 (October 2014): 766–74. doi: 10.2519/jospt.2014.5575.

Luedke, Lace E., et al. "Influence of Step Rate on Shin Injury and Anterior Knee Pain in High School Runners." *Medicine and Science in Sports and Exercise* 48, no. 7 (2016): 1244–50. doi: 10.1249/MSS.0000000000000890.

Malisoux, Laurent, et al. "Can Parallel Use of Different Running Shoes Decrease Running-Related Injury Risk?" *Scandinavian Journal of Medicine and Science in Sports* 25, no. 1 (February 2015): 110–15. doi: 10.1111/sms.12154.

———. "Injury Risk in Runners Using Standard or Motion Control Shoes: A Randomised Controlled Trial with Participant and Assessor Blinding." *British Journal of Sports Medicine* 50, no. 8 (January 2016). doi: 10.1136/ bjsports-2015-095031.

Mann, Robert, et al. "Fluctuations in Strike Index and Spatiotemporal Parameters in Previously Injured Versus Uninjured Runners." *British Journal of Sports Medicine* 48, no. 7 (2014): 632–33. doi: 10.1136/bjsports-2014-093494.

McCallion, Ciara, et al. "Acute Differences in Foot Strike and Spatiotemporal Variables for Shod, Barefoot or Minimalist Male Runners." *Journal of Sports Science and Medicine* 13, no. 2 (May 2014): 280–86.

McKeon, Patrick O., et al. "The Foot Core System: A New Paradigm for Understanding Intrinsic Foot Muscle Function." *British Journal of Sports Medicine* 49, no. 5 (2015): 290. doi:10.1136/bjsports-2013-092690.

Meira, Erik P., and Jason Brumitt. "Influence of the Hip on Patients with Patellofemoral Pain Syndrome: A Systematic Review." *Sports Health* 3, no. 5 (September 2011): 455–65. doi: 10.1177/1941738111415006.

Mientjes, Martine, and Martyn Shorten. "Contoured Cushioning: Effects of Surface Compressibility and Curvature on Heel Pressure Distribution." *Journal of Footwear Science* 3, no. 1 (2011). doi:10.1080/19424280.2010.536587.

Moore, S., et al. "Effects of Neck Posture on Ventilation and Perceived Exertion in Trained Females." *International Journal of Exercise Science* 8, no. 2 (2014): Article 38. http://digitalcommons.wku.edu/ijesab/vol8/iss2/38.

Nelson, Richard C., and Robert J. Gregor. "Biomechanics of Distance Running: A Longitudinal Study. *Research Quarterly* 47, no. 3 (October 1976): 417–28.

Nigg, Benno M. "The Role of Impact Forces and Foot Pronation: A New Paradigm." *Clinical Journal of Sports Medicine* 11, no. 1 (January 2001): 2–9.

Nigg, Benno M., et al. "Running Shoes and Running Injuries: Mythbusting and a Proposal for Two New Paradigms: Preferred Movement Path and Comfort Filter." *British Journal of Sports Medicine* (2015). doi: 10.1136/bjsports-2015-095054.

Nigg, Benno M., and Hendrick Enders. "Barefoot Running—Some Critical Considerations." *Footwear Science* 5, no. 1 (2013): 1–7. doi: 10.1080/19424280.2013.766649.

Noehren, Brian, Irene Davis, and Joseph Hamill. "Prospective Study of the Biomechanical Factors Associated with Iliotibial Band Syndrome." *Clinical Biomechanics* 22 (2007): 951–56.

Peters, Jeroen S., and Natalie L. Tyson. "Proximal Exercises Are Effective in Treating Patellofemoral Pain Syndrome: A Systematic Review." *International Journal of Sports Physical Therapy* 8, no. 5 (2013): 689–700.

Robinson, R. L. and Robert J. Nee. "Analysis of Hip Strength in Females Seeking Physical Therapy Treatment for Unilateral Patellofemoral Pain Syndrome." *Journal of Orthopedic Sports Physical Therapy* 37, no. 5 (May 2007): 232–38.

Saunders, Philo U., et al. "Factors Affecting Running Economy in Trained Distance Runners." *Sports Medicine* 34, no. 7 (2004): 465–85.

Selkowitz, D. M., G. J. Beneck, and C. M. Powers. "Which Exercises Target the Gluteal Muscles While Minimizing Activation of the Tensor Fascia Lata? Electromyographic Assessment Using Fine-Wire Electrodes." *Journal of Orthopaedic & Sports Physical Therapy* 43, no. 2 (February 2013): 54–64. doi: 10.2519/jospt.2013.4116.

Shorten, Martyn. "The Energetics of Running and Running Shoes." *Journal of Biomechanics* 26, supplement 1 (1993): 41–51.

Shorten, Martyn, and Martine Mientjes. "The 'Heel Impact' Force Peak During Running Is Neither 'Heel' Nor 'Impact' and Does Not Quantify Shoe Cushioning Effects." *Journal of Footwear Science* 3, no. 1 (February 13, 2011). doi: 10.1080/19424280.2010.542186.

Simic, L., N. Sarabon, and Goran Markovic. "Does Pre-Exercise Static Stretching Inhibit Maximal Muscular Performance? A Meta-Analytical Review." *Scandinavian Journal of Medicine and Science in Sports* 23, no. 2 (March 2013): 131–48. doi: 10.1111/j.1600-0838.2012.01444.x.

Stearne, Sarah M., et al. "The Foot's Arch and the Energetics of Human Locomotion." *Scientific Reports* 6, article number 19403 (January 2016). doi:10.1038/srep19403.

Tung, K. D., et al. "A Test of the Metabolic Cost of Cushioning Hypothesis During Unshod and Shod Running." *Medicine and Science in Sports and Exercise* 46, no. 2 (February 2014): 324–29. doi: 10.1249/MSS.0b013e3182a63b81.

Willson, John D., et al. "Short Term Changes in Running Mechanics and Footwear Strike Pattern After Introduction to Minimalistic Footwear." *PM&R Journal* 6, no. 1 (2014): 34–43. doi: http://dx.doi.org/10.1016/j.pmrj.2013.08.602.

Willy, Richard W., and Irene S. Davis. "Kinematic and Kinetic Comparison of Running in Standard and Minimalist Shoes." *Medicine & Science in Sports & Exercise* 46, no. 2 (February 2014): 318–323. doi: 10.1249/MSS.0b013e3182a595d2 Applied Sciences.

Willy, Richard W., et al. "Mirror Gait Retraining for the Treatment of Patellofemoral Pain in Female Runners." *Clinical Biomechanics* 27, no. 10 (December 2012): 1045–51.

WEBSITE ARTICLES

Bartold, Simon. "Gait Analysis: How Should We Run? Will Gait Retraining Help?" Bartoldbiomechanics.com, May 2016. https://www.bartoldbiomechanics.com/articles/gait-analysis.

Brooks Running, white paper. "Stride Signature: An Individual's Unique Running Form Defined by the Body's Habitual Motion Path." 2014. http://www.ebooks10.com/read-books/2014/05/157276550/brooks-stride-signature.html.

Burfoot, Amby. "How Much Should You Lean for Optimal Running Form? Two New Studies Show a Slight Forward Posture May Help You Run More Economically." Runnersworld.com, June 29, 2016. http://www.runnersworld.com/general-interest/how-much-should-you-lean-for-optimal-running-form.

Fitzgerald, Matt. "Q&A: An In-Depth Look at Better Running Form," Competitor.com, April 4, 2014. http://running.competitor.com/2014/04/training/qa-an-in-depth-look-at-better-running-form_10054#8dCHitmVrUCbGlip.99.

Goom, Tom. "Gluteus Medius—Evidence Based Rehab," Running-physio.com, May 8, 2012. http://www.running-physio.com/glutemed/.

Hughes, Marty. "Six Reasons to Realign the Big Toe." Naturalfootgear.com, 2015. http://naturalfootgear.com/blogs/education/17914716-six-reasons-to-realign-the-big-toe?mc_cid=43995396b2&mc_eid=a10b37076e.

Hutchinson, Alex. "The Problem with 180 Strides per Minute: Some Personal Data." *Sweat Science,* September 8, 2011. http://sweatscience.com/the-problem-with-180-strides-per-minute-some-personal-data/.

Jones, Brett. "Best Thoracic Mobility Exercise—The "Brettzel" Stretch." https://www.youtube.com/watch?v=yMnamNJZMBk.

ABOUT THE AUTHOR

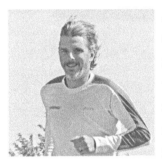

JONATHAN BEVERLY WAS THE EDITOR IN CHIEF of *Running Times* magazine from 2000 to 2015. During those years, he wrote a popular monthly editor's note, more than 35 feature stories, and dozens of training articles, athlete profiles, race reports, and shoe and gear reviews. Prior to becoming editor, Jonathan wrote regularly as a freelancer while directing international exchange programs for universities. He has run 26 marathons and hundreds of road and trail races throughout the world and has coached adult runners and junior high and high school track and cross-country. He lives on the border of Nebraska and Colorado.

INDEX

Boldface page references denote illustrations. <u>Underscored</u> page references denote boxed text.

H

Hallelujah drill, 194–95
Hamstrings
  injury from
    increasing cadence, 113
    tight hips, 39
  lunging lizard stretch for,
    46, **46**
Hands, 74, 76–77
Harness, climbing, 192–93
Head position, 90–93
  exercises, 92–93
  forward-head posture, 91–92
Heel strike, 13–21, 108
High knees, 139, **139**
Hip extension, 36, 40
  action plan for, 198
  glute tests
    pigeon hip extension, 56, **56**
    standing hip extension, 57,
      57
  improving glute strength, 53
  performance linked to, 58
  shoulder issues and, 76
  during sleep, 166–67
Hip extension stretch, 37, 42
Hip extension test, **36**, 36–37
Hip flexibility, working on, 153–54
Hip flexion, 35–36
Hip flexors
  lack of elastically loading, 40
  releasing, 58
  stretching, 25, 41–52
    active isolated quad stretch,
      48–49, **49**
    the Brettzel, 48
    couch stretch, 47, **47**
    kneeling hip flexor stretch, **42**,
      42–43
    leg swing, 50, **50**
    lunging lizard, 46, **46**
    Running Warrior, 45, **45**
    self-massage, 52, **52**
    single-leg squat with stretch, **49**,
      49–50
    during sleep, 167
    standing hip stretch, 44, **44**
    walking lunge, 51, **51**
  tight, 37–41
    dynamic stretches for, 48–52
    forward rotation of hips with, 39
    injury associated with, 38–39
    sitting effect on, 38
    static stretches for, 41–48
Hip flick, 59
Hips, 23–34
  bowl/bucket, 29–30, **30**
  flexibility in, 25, 37–42
  forward rotation with tight hip
    flexors, 39
  injury associated with weak, 24
  pelvic proprioception, 27–29
  rotating, 25, 30–31
  sitting position, 35, **35**
  stacked under torso, 28–30
  stretching, 25, 41–52, 166, 198

I

Iliotibial (IT) band syndrome, 24, 66,
  108
Inflexibilities, created by lifestyle, 26
Injury
  acceptance of, 156–57
  decrease with
    faster cadence, 116
    reduced braking, 58
    shoe variety, 186
    tight hip flexors, 38–39
    training variability, 126–27
    weak glutes, 39, 66
  hamstring from
    increasing cadence, 113
    tight hips, 39
  increase with
    hip weakness, 24
    lower cadence, 108, 110
    plyometrics, 59
  mismatch diseases, 7
  overuse, 127
  prevention and strength, 150
  pronation and, 171–72, 174
  repetitive stress, 127
Injury proofing, 157
Insanity, defined, 156
Inspiration, 197

Integrative wall push-off, 90, **90**
IT band syndrome, 24, 66, 108

J

Jump squat, <u>59</u>, 64, **64**

K

Kinesthetic awareness, 168
Kinetic chain, 23
Kneeling hip flexor stretch, **42**,
    42–43

L

Landing. *See also* Foot strike
    cadence and, 108
    overstriding, 26
Landing zone, 13–21
Lats
    doorway lat stretch, 85, **85**
    foam roller lat release, 86, **86**
    lat stretch with roller, 84, **84**
    tight, 84
Lat stretch with roller, 84, **84**
Lean
    cadence and, 122
    forward, 32–33, 190–91
Leg swing, 50, **50**
Loading, 112
Lumo Run, 124
Lunge-balance sequence, **142–43**,
    142–44, 161
Lunge matrix, **137**, 137–38, 159–60
Lunging lizard, 46, **46**

M

Marching bridge, 61, **61**
Maximum speed, 134
Mental release of running, 146
Metabolic cost, 114, 152
Midfoot strike, 13–21
Midrun striders, 193–94

Minimalism, 13–14, 113, 135, 170, 175,
    184
Mismatch diseases, 7
Mobility
    integrating work into everyday life,
        161–67, 198
    perils of sitting, 35–52
    restriction of, 9, 42, 52
    shoulders, 80–86, **82**
    stretches for (*see* Stretches)
Motion-control shoes, 171–74, 177
Motivation, 154–55
Movement pattern/path, 44
    changing cadence to create new,
        117–18
    changing shoes and, 133
    drills for new, 133–34
    plasticity, 126
    preferred, 5–9, 125–26
        flowing water analogy, 9
        improving, 8
        limits to, 6–8
        shoes and, 173, 175, 179
    retraining, 26–27
    variability, 126–32
    walking, 120
Movement signature, 5
Multitasking, 161–67
Muscle atrophy, 7, 26, 97
Muscles, shortened, 7
Muscular recruitment patterns,
    152
Myths, 1–11

N

Neck
    exercises, 92–93
    posture, 92
Neutral position, rotating hips into,
    <u>25</u>, 30–31
Neutral posture, 30–31, 34

O

Overpronation, 171–74
Overrotation, 39

Stretches *(cont.)*
    static, 41–48
        the Brettzel, 48
        couch stretch, 47, **47**
        kneeling hip flexor stretch, **42**,
          42–43
        lunging lizard, 46, **46**
        Running Warrior, 45, **45**
        standing hip stretch, 44, **44**
Stride
    failure of shoes to change, 175–76
    shaking up yours, 130–32
    shifting your stride, 197
    steps to reclaiming, 25
Stride length
    cadence and, 105–6
    maintaining, 106
    overstriding, 106, 108, 116
    for speed, 58
Strides, 134–36
Stride signature, 3–4, 73
Stryd power meter, 124

T

Terrain, varying, 129–32, 197
Time management
    integrating elements into process,
      161
    making elements mandatory, 159–61
    multitasking, 161–67
Toebox, shoe, 184–86
Toe curls, 103–4, **103–4**
Toes, splaying of, 99–100
Toe spreader, plastic, 100
Toe yoga, 100–101, 166
Towel pull, 103, **103**
Transversus abdominis, 70–71, 164
Turnover. *See* Cadence

U

Ultimate Frisbee, 131

V

Variability, 125–44
    action plan, 197–98
    changing shoes, 133
    drills for new movement pattern,
      133–34
      A-Skip, 140, **140**
      backward running, 141
      barefoot strides, 135–36
      butt kick, 140, **140**
      carioca, 141, **141**
      high knees, 139, **139**
      lunge-balance sequence,
        142–43, 142–44
      lunge matrix, **137**, 137–38
      single-leg balance, **136**,
        136–37
      strides, 134–36
    injury protection with, 126–27
    plasticity, 129
    ruts, 126–28, 197
    terrain, 129–32, 197
Vertical compression test, 28, **28**
Visualization form cues,
    192–93

W

Walking lunge, 51, **51**
Walking muscle patterns, 120
Wall test, Wharton, 91–92
Wharton open arm stretch, 86–87, **87**
Wharton shoulder stretch, 87–88, **88**